HOW TO BECOME
A VETERINARIAN

*Find Out How To Start a Career
Working With Animals & Discover
If It's The Right Job For You!*

By

Karen Wilson

TABLE OF CONTENTS

INTRODUCTION

The average person assumes that veterinarians choose this field because of their love for animals. They are only half correct, at least as far as I am concerned. I chose this field because I wanted to be able to help pets *and* their people. Even though I mostly treat dogs and cats, I love almost every other species of animal. I love meeting new people and talking about how we share the same love for animals. I have a passion for all things medicine, and I also enjoy teaching and sharing my medical knowledge. If I get to do these things every day while snuggling the occasional puppy or kitten, who am I to complain?

But the life of a veterinarian isn't as simple as doing all the things that I love every minute of the day. There are moments that are stressful like when someone's Chihuahua is coming in as an emergency because he can't breathe. There are immensely sad moments like when someone is saying goodbye to their feline friend of fifteen years. Yet even in those difficult times, the silver lining is that I helped a pet in an awful situation, and I alleviated someone's stress and grief. It takes a lot of energy to go through these scenarios. It happens at least once a week for me, but I have some colleagues in the field who go through it almost daily.

Despite some of the lows that come with this job, there are many highs, and that's just part of what makes the work worthwhile. For many of us, being a veterinarian is a very rewarding career because you can make a world of difference in the lives of the pets and people that you meet. You can inspire those around you, and there is always new information about the ways to practice medicine. Life is rarely dull when you're a veterinarian!

If you've ever thought about becoming a veterinarian, or if you're just curious about what it takes to become one, this book is for you! There are actually many options for you when deciding how to utilize your veterinary medical degree, more than just work in a general practicing clinic for dogs and cats. In addition to discussing some of the ins and outs of veterinary medicine, I will describe the journey leading up to admission into a veterinary school, how life in veterinary school plays out, and what to expect once you've graduated. It can be a humbling yet exciting experience!

CHAPTER 1:

WHAT IS A VETERINARIAN?

A veterinarian is a type of medical doctor that specializes in the diagnosis and treatment of illnesses that affect animals. They ensure the health and well-being of animals while also ensuring the health of the general public. This is because there are certain diseases and parasites that can be transmitted from animals to people, creating a public health risk.

Most general practicing veterinarians (like me) work in a clinical or hospital setting. During the daytime, we see scheduled appointments for preventive care services and medical issues. Some clinics may operate on a walk-in basis like vaccine clinics or emergency rooms, though there may be some days where even a general practicing vet needs to help an emergency that suddenly shows up in the lobby.

Veterinarians are trained to help combat infectious diseases, and routine vaccinations are an important part of disease prevention. The average dog and cat should receive specific vaccines once a year with the exception of the rabies vaccine, which can be given every three years in certain cases. Veterinarians must also ensure that pets are free from parasites because certain skin mites and intestinal parasites can make people ill.

Veterinarians in general practice can also treat common illnesses. Ear infections and skin infections occur quite often. External parasites like fleas and mites can cause these kinds of infections. Environmental allergies and food allergies can also trigger these kinds of problems. Pets with ear and skin problems can be very uncomfortable. Another common health problem is gastrointestinal upset. Dogs and cats with GI problems often present with vomiting, diarrhea, or both. Veterinarians are able to evaluate these pets and try to determine what caused it as well as how best to treat the issue.

Spaying and neutering are also part of a veterinarian's role, especially if they work in general practice or in animal shelters. These two surgeries involve the removal of specific organs so that animals cannot reproduce. Research shows that routine spays and neuters have decreased pet overpopulation, thus reducing the number of dogs and cats who are euthanized in shelters each year.

In some cases, a general practicing vet can also perform some uncommon surgical procedures like skin tumor removals. For more complicated procedures, there are veterinarians who specialize in certain departments, and general vets can refer patients to these specialty vets. There are also veterinarians who specialize in emergency medicine and critical care. Veterinarians can also have jobs outside of clinical practice, which we will discuss in later sections of this book.

One of the most important duties of being a veterinarian is client education. In the age of the internet and "Dr. Google," there is a lot of misinformation that exists in various websites and forums. Some of this misinformation can be very dangerous! It is our job to communicate complicated medical information in a way that the average pet owner can understand. We must also share knowledge about health risks that can impact their pet's health *and* their own health.

CHAPTER 2:

HOW DOES VETERINARY MEDICINE COMPARE TO HUMAN MEDICINE?

Veterinary medicine is very similar to human medicine. Veterinarians go to school for the same length of time as human physicians. After graduating high school, you are encouraged to obtain some education in college before applying to a veterinary school. Not all vet schools require this, but most of the schools in the United States require certain prerequisite courses at the college level before you apply to vet school.

Once in veterinary school, students are taught about normal anatomy and how various parts of the body work when healthy. These are subjects such as neurology (the study of the nervous system), cardiology (the study of the cardiovascular system), endocrinology (the study of endocrine glands and hormones), and dermatology (the study of skin). These are just some of the areas of study. In fact, there is really only one area of study that is different from human medicine: anatomy and physiology.

For most veterinary students, anatomy class starts with a discussion about dogs. Early on, the class starts with external structures and then moves internally over the coming weeks. Even though there are some obvious differences between dogs and humans, the names for a majority of body parts, organs, blood vessels, and nerves are exactly the same as the names used for human body parts. For example, the thigh bone in humans is called a femur, and that's exactly what we call it in veterinary medicine.

Once students have studied the dog, they go on to study the cat and the structural differences between the two. For large animal anatomy, students learn about the horse. This is where anatomy class gets a little complicated, because the horse has very different limbs and a gastrointestinal tract that is very unlike that of dogs and cats. For students interested in exotics and other animals, there are even *more* body parts to learn!

All veterinary students must pass a rigorous board exam before they can practice medicine. Once they graduate, some new veterinarians decide to go into practice right away. If the new graduate is looking for some more experience before practicing by themselves, they may choose to complete an internship for a year or two. If a newly graduated veterinarian is looking to become board certified in a certain specialty, that internship is followed up with a residency for a few years. Just like in human medicine, a board exam is necessary upon completion of the residency.

Veterinarians can practice medicine in clinics, hospitals, or mobile practices. Many of the same principles of human medicine apply in veterinary practices, but emergency veterinary medicine is very different. For instance, there are no emergency responder or ambulance services that are funded by the government. Some ambulance services exist in a few areas, but these are private businesses run by veterinarians or veterinary professionals. Emergency animal hospitals are also businesses, and so payment is typically due right away. If you injure yourself and need to go to the emergency room, the government provides funding that allows most citizens to receive treatment without having to pay ahead of time. Unfortunately, this is not the case in veterinary medicine.

One of the best things about veterinary medicine is that we share a lot of scientific information with our human medicine colleagues and vice versa. Many of the clinical trials that are used for the development of treatments in human medicine utilize rodents as the subjects. This is because mice and rats are similar to humans both genetically and biologically. They even age the same way that we do, but because their life expectancies are shorter, we can study things faster than we can in humans.

Sometimes, veterinarians can borrow techniques from human medicine. One great example is how we use certain aspects of integrative medicine for animals. Integrative medicine is a holistic approach to healing. Acupuncture, which is the use of small needles placed in certain locations on the body to promote healing, was first used in humans thousands of years ago. It may surprise you to know that we can perform acupuncture for animals, and it works well in many cases! Horses, cats, and dogs greatly benefit from acupuncture for many health problems such as arthritis or joint pain.

There are many medications in human medicine that we use for animals. Many of the antibiotics and supplements used in people are also prescribed for dogs and cats. This also applies to anxiety medications and some pain relievers like opioids. However, there are some human medications that are extremely dangerous for animals. Non-steroidal anti-inflammatories (NSAIDs) like ibuprofen and Naproxen can cause severe bleeding and kidney failure in dogs and cats, even if very small quantities are ingested.

Much of the equipment used in both fields of medicine may come from the same medical distributor. The surgical supplies and suture materials used in veterinary medicine are also used by human surgeons. Some of the dental equipment used for dental prophylaxes and tooth extractions are identical to the tools used by human dentists. I've seen this firsthand because the ultrasonic scaler at my dental hygienist's clinic is the exact same model that I use at the veterinary hospital where I work.

CHAPTER 3:

WHAT KINDS OF ANIMALS DO VETERINARIANS WORK WITH?

The average veterinarian has a set number of species with whom they work. It can be difficult for a human physician to know everything about just one species, so you can imagine that having to learn about multiple species can be even more challenging.

Most small animal veterinarians like myself focus on the practice of medicine for dogs and cats. There may be some practices that just focus on dogs or on cats, the latter of which has its benefits because most cats prefer peace and quiet rather than having to listen to barking, excitable dogs in the hospital lobby. Some small animal practices may have the ability to work with "pocket pets," a term that applies to common pet store animals like small lizards, birds, rodents, rabbits, and guinea pigs. There are even a few that have experience dealing with pot-bellied pigs!

Large animal practices focus on horses and common farm animals like cattle, goats, pigs, and sheep. In some cases, pot-bellied pigs can also fall into this category. Large animal practices are different from small animal hospitals because while most small animal vets operate in a standalone building or clinic, large animal vets seldom work this way. Many large animal vets are considered "mobile" practices because they often have to drive great distances to see their patients, especially if an owner has no way of transporting their large cow or horse.

There are some veterinarians who only work with food animals. This is similar to being a large animal veterinarian because pigs and cattle fall into his category, and chickens are also cared for by food animal vets. The vet's job is to make sure that these animals are being provided good sources of food, water, and clean shelters. They must also ensure that they stay healthy and receive vaccinations. If food animals become sick, veterinarians must be careful to only use medications that are safe for human consumption. Besides meat, food animal vets also ensure that the eggs, milk, and butter that we eat come from healthy animals.

Zoo animal veterinarians are the superstars of the veterinary world because they see *hundreds* of different animal species every day! If you've ever been to a zoo, you probably saw lots of different animals, from lions and panthers to bears, birds, reptiles, amphibians, and small rodents. The average day of a zoo animal vet is always exciting and different, but there is also difficulty in the fact that no two days are the same! There are so many subtle rules that apply. For example, you have to remember which medications are dangerous to use for certain animals, and you need to be able to calculate drug dosages for patients who weigh anywhere from 300 grams to 300 pounds!

Aquatic veterinarians work with marine animals and invertebrates. Fish, sea turtles, seals, sharks, dolphins, and whales are just a few examples of the diverse species that the average aquatic vet will work with each day. Aquatic vets ensure the health and safety of marine animals, and they can perform many of the same treatments and procedures that regular vets can. Animals who live inside of aquariums, oceanariums, and marine life centers are cared for by aquatic veterinarians. Aquatic vets also see to the medical needs of marine wildlife and play a major role in conservation efforts.

CHAPTER 4:

WHAT KINDS OF VETERINARIANS ARE THERE?

There are many different types of jobs available for veterinarians. The majority of veterinarians practice medicine in a clinical setting. This means that they work in a clinic or a hospital location, examining and treating their patients every day. For large animal, zoo, and aquatic vets, the definition of a clinical setting can be very different because medicine is sometimes practiced in the field instead of in a physical building.

Small animal veterinarians

Small animal practice makes up the biggest percentage of veterinarians in the United States. Many of them focus on the care of cats and dogs. The average small animal practice will see both dogs and cats, though there are some "cat only" practices that can cater to the needs of frightened felines. Also referred to as companion animal practices, some small animal practices may see rodents, rabbits, birds, reptiles, and other exotic or "pocket pets," depending on the vet's experience working with these species.

Preventive care is one of the main offerings in small animal practice. Routine vaccinations to prevent against certain bacterial and viral infections are important, especially when the infections are highly contagious and/or sometimes fatal. The rabies virus, for example, is transmitted when an infected animal bites a dog or cat. If a rabies infection occurs, there is no cure. Rabies is 100 percent fatal to the pet who develops it, and it puts humans at risk because it can be transmitted to us if we are bitten by an infected animal. For this reason, rabies virus is a major public health concern, and almost all 50 states require dogs and cats to receive a routine rabies vaccine.

The prevention of parasites is also an important job for small animal vets. Routine deworming can prevent illness in pets *and* in people. For example, dogs and cats can pick up intestinal parasites like roundworms and hookworms from the feces of an infected animal. When these worms get into the gastrointestinal tract, they can cause vomiting, diarrhea, and weight loss. If humans contact infected fecal material and don't practice good hygiene (e.g. washing their hands), they can become infected. Hookworms are one of the worst kinds because they can migrate to the skin or to the eyes. This is called cutaneous and ocular larva migrans, respectively. The ocular form of the disease can cause vision loss.

External parasites can also be a problem. Fleas and mites are small bugs that can live on the skin of a dog or cat. These parasites can cause itchiness and skin infection. In severe cases, fleas can cause life-threatening blood loss and can transmit bacteria that cause fever and illness. Certain mites like scabies can jump from pets to people and cause intense itchy skin. Ticks are another small bug that can bite our pets, but the tick only jumps on for feeding purposes. Males may stick around for a while, but females leave to go lay their eggs. Like other external parasites, ticks can carry bacterial diseases that can make dogs and cats very sick. Most veterinarians carry topical or oral flea and tick preventives that pets should receive all year round.

Most small animal vets can perform routine surgery. Spaying and neutering are common surgeries that are performed under general anesthesia. This means that the patient is completely unconscious so that they can remain still for the procedure while experiencing no pain. Spaying and neutering involves the surgical removal of specific reproductive organs: a male's testicles are removed during a neuter, and a female's ovaries and uterus are removed during a spay. There is currently some debate about the right age to perform this surgery. For vets in an animal shelter setting, it is ideal to spay and neuter as soon as possible, which may mean that a puppy or a kitten will have surgery before they are adopted. Some vets feel there may be some benefit to waiting until a pet is fully grown before performing surgery. Current evidence suggests that somewhere in the middle, about five to six months of age, may be better for most cats and dogs.

Some small animal vets can perform dental procedures for their patients. Dental health is important because animals use their mouths for so many different functions, not just for chewing! Brushing is just as beneficial to them as it is for us, but without routine dental care, periodontal disease can develop. Most adult dogs and cats should have a deep tooth cleaning (dental prophylaxis) with their vet at least once a year. Dental cleanings of this nature should also be performed under general anesthesia because it is not possible to clean below the gumline when a dog or cat is awake, no matter how nicely you ask them!

Besides preventive medicine, most dog and cat owners bring their pets to the vet when there are signs of illness. Some of the most common presenting complaints are vomiting, diarrhea, lethargy, itchy skin or ears, coughing, sneezing, and lack of appetite. When sick pets come to see their doctor, it is important to ask if the owner is seeing any of these clinical signs. A thorough medical history is the best way for a veterinarian to figure out what their patient's problem might be.

Diagnostics are a key factor in determining the diagnosis for a sick patient. Most small animal vets are able to run blood samples through a machine in their hospital. These blood analyzers can tell you if there is a problem with the function of the internal organs or the pet's immune system. Urine samples can also be analyzed to look for evidence of infection or problems with the kidneys. Some small animal practices may have access to special imaging tests like x-rays and ultrasound, which are ways that vets can take pictures of the insides of a patient. There may be other diagnostics at a vet's disposal, but for more specialized testing, sometimes samples are sent to reference laboratories for more information.

Small animal hospitals are also equipped for treating very sick and critical patients. Dehydrated patients may need to have intravenous fluids delivered continuously, and patients who are having breathing problems from pneumonia or heart disease may need to recover in an oxygen cage. If multiple medications are necessary, or if some medications need to be delivered via an injection, veterinary nurses can administer these while a patient is hospitalized.

Sadly, there may be situations where a pet's illness cannot be cured, or a pet may have a poor quality of life due to pain and suffering. Veterinarians are trained to perform humane euthanasia, which is the administration of an overdose of anesthetic drugs, causing the heart to stop. It is not a painful procedure, and while it is often difficult to say goodbye to a beloved furry family member, it is always the last kind thing that we can do for them.

Dental specialists

Even though most small animal veterinarians can perform basic dental procedures like cleanings and extractions, there are some situations that call for more complicated techniques.

Veterinary dentists or dental specialists can see patients who are referred to them.

Cats can develop some serious dental disease. There are cavity-like holes in teeth called resorptive lesions that can occur when the immune system attacks the tooth. Researchers aren't sure why this happens, but they know that diseased teeth, teeth with dental tartar, and the presence of gingivitis can increase the risk of tooth resorption. When there are many resorptive lesions or severe generalized inflammation of the gums (called gingivostomatitis), all of the teeth will need to be extracted in order to minimize inflammation and provide comfort. When all teeth are extracted, this is called a full mouth extraction or FME. Dental specialists are well trained in the removal of these diseased teeth.

Dogs can also develop severe dental disease, and there are some dogs who may benefit from full mouth extractions. Dogs can also go to the dentist if they have misaligned teeth. Dentists can create doggie braces to realign the teeth, or they can perform crown amputations to shorten the height of the teeth, minimizing trauma to the palate or the tongue. Fractured teeth can be treated via techniques like vital pulpotomy or root canal therapy, just like in people. To protect working dogs like canine police officers from fracturing their teeth on the job, dentists can reinforce their teeth with titanium crowns.

Soft tissue surgery

The average general practicing small animal vet is trained to perform spay and neuter surgeries. These are known as soft tissue surgeries because they involve pretty much any surgical procedure that doesn't involve bone. Some small animal vets can perform non-routine soft tissue surgeries such as mass removals and skin tag removals. In emergency situations, some can perform Cesarean sections (the surgical removal of puppies or kittens when a laboring mom is having birthing difficulties) or emergency spay procedures. An emergency spay is indicated when a pyometra is present. This is when a female dog's or cat's uterus fills up with pus. Pyometra is a life-threatening emergency where surgery is needed right away.

Depending on the vet's comfort level, they may also be able to remove a ruptured spleen in an emergency situation. The spleen is an organ that stores red blood cells and plays a role in your dog's or cat's immune system. Tumors can grow on the spleen and rupture. Another splenic trauma situation is when a patient is hit by a car, or the spleen can become entrapped when a deep-chested or large breed dog develops bloat. In certain situations, a dog's stomach can fill with air or fluid, and then the stomach rotates on itself, causing a condition known as gastric dilatation volvulus. This is a life-threatening emergency that can be fatal in just a few hours.

There may be some vets who are not comfortable with surgery or have not had prior experience performing certain procedures. General practicing vets can refer their patients to specialty vets who have had extra training to become boarded soft tissue surgeons. Besides procedures that general practicing vets can perform, soft tissue surgeons have experience with invasive and difficult surgeries. For example, there are some cases where a dog's lung lobe needs to be removed. This may be due to trauma, torsion, or the presence of a lung tumor in that lobe. To get to the affected lobe, the dog's chest will need to be opened. This complicates things because dogs cannot breathe with an open chest, so a ventilator is necessary to help with breathing while the surgeon works to perform this very technical procedure. Complications can occur such as bleeding during and after the surgery, so it is best to have a surgeon who has experience and special training with this type of procedure.

Orthopedic surgery

Orthopedic surgery involves working with bony tissues instead of soft tissues. Just like in people, the skeleton of a dog or cat or horse is made up of solid bone. To help keep bones together, there are bands of connective tissue called tendons and ligaments. These bands stretch across the surface of two or more bones to form a joint space. Animals with joint and bone problems will sometimes need to be seen by an orthopedic specialist if treatment is beyond the scope of what a general practicing vet can do.

In small animal veterinary medicine, pets may need to see a specialist if they have a bone fracture from falling or getting hit by a car. With simple fractures (only one clean break in a bone), some vets can help them heal by placing a splint or a cast around the broken bone. If the fracture is more complicated (e.g., there are many pieces, or the fracture is in a place that cannot be splinted), surgical repair may be necessary. Pets are placed under general anesthesia so the orthopedic surgeon can use metal plates and screws to put the bone back together.

In human medicine, a person can injure an important ligament called the anterior cruciate ligament or ACL. This is located in a person's knee. Dogs have a similar ligament in their knees, but we call it the cranial cruciate ligament or CCL. When a dog injures his CCL, his knee becomes unstable. The shin bone or tibia will shift forward as he steps, causing intense pain. Special surgical techniques are utilized to stabilize the joint so that the bone does not shift forward, thus relieving pain and minimizing arthritis.

There are certain situations where a broken bone cannot be repaired. This may be due to the severity of the break or because something like an aggressive bone cancer has caused the bone to fracture. In these situations, a limb amputation is necessary. This is when the surgeon removes the entire affected limb while the pet is under general anesthesia. While this sounds like an intense way to treat a bone problem, it has great benefits for the pet. Dogs and cats tend to quickly learn how to walk on three legs instead of four, and the cause of their severe pain is removed once surgery is complete. Larger animals like horses are usually not good candidates for limb amputation surgery due to their size, but they can still undergo orthopedic surgery for other problems like fractures and joint disease.

Cardiology

A specialist who focuses on the diagnosis and treatment of heart diseases in animals is called a veterinary cardiologist. The heart is one of the most important organs in the body. It is constantly pumping blood cells which carry oxygen to the entire body. Without oxygen, the body cannot function. Sometimes there are problems where the rhythm by which the heart pumps is irregular. The heart's electrical activity misfires, and it cannot pump blood the way it normally would. In other situations, the heart may pump too quickly or too slowly, or it develops problems where the chambers of the heart cannot fill and pump enough blood to meet oxygen demands. Heart disease can cause coughing, weakness, exercise intolerance, collapse, and sometimes death.

DOG HEART ANATOMY

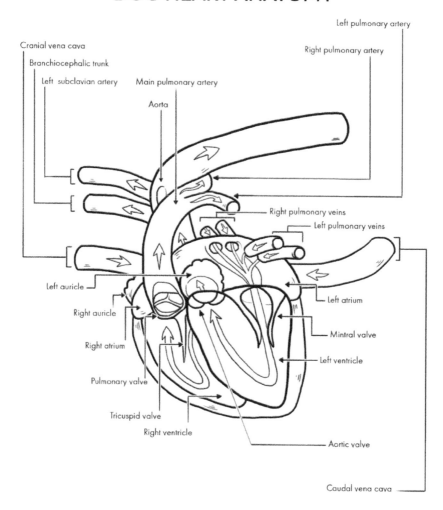

When heart disease is suspected, some general practicing vets can recommend testing to help determine the cause. They can check the blood pressure of their patient, and they can check the heart's rhythm with a test called an electrocardiogram (or ECG). Sometimes an x-ray of the chest can show if the heart is enlarged or if there is a problem with the lungs and the blood vessels around the heart. An ultrasound of the heart (called an echocardiogram) can allow the vet to look inside the chambers of the heart, to assess the valves between the chambers, and to see if the walls of the heart are too thick or too thin. Because this information can be complicated, or if there is a situation where open-heart surgery is necessary, the patient will need to go see a veterinary cardiologist.

There are many different medications that cardiologists can prescribe. Some of them are blood pressure medications that widen blood vessels, making it easier for the heart to pump blood. Other medications can help restore the heartbeat to a normal rhythm. If there is fluid building up in the abdomen or around the lungs due to heart failure, diuretic medications can help remove excess fluid from the body.

Heart surgery may be necessary in certain situations. For example, a dog with a large number of heartworms (a parasite that lives inside of the heart and main pulmonary artery) may need to have these worms surgically removed if he develops a problem called caval syndrome. Inherited conditions that affect the heart valves like pulmonic stenosis and patent ductus arteriosus require heart surgery to be fixed. In conditions where the heart rate is dangerously low, a pacemaker can be surgically placed to help maintain a normal rhythm.

In horses, atrial fibrillation is one of the most common heart arrhythmias. Atrial fibrillation can be due to underlying heart enlargement or can be present without underlying disease. Veterinary cardiologists can sometimes correct this with medication, but if there is no response, they can attempt transvenous electrical cardioversion while the horse is under general anesthesia. This involves the use of electrodes and a cardiac defibrillator to help shock the heart back into a normal rhythm.

Dermatology

There are also veterinary specialists who focus on the diagnosis and treatment of skin diseases. These doctors are known as veterinary dermatologists. Most dermatological illnesses will affect the ears, skin, and sometimes the mouth and paws. In some cases, underlying hormonal diseases like diabetes mellitus and Cushing's disease can cause skin and ear issues. Veterinary dermatologists can help.

Skin and ear problems are common issues that the average general practicing vet may address, but for those who suffer from chronic ear infections and chronic skin infections, the dermatologist may be able to do more. Allergies are one of the biggest causes of ear and skin problems. Dermatologists can perform intradermal skin testing to determine which allergens are causing the patient's clinical signs. Then the allergens can be put into a vaccine that is made specifically for the patient. This is called immunotherapy. It is a way to "reboot" the immune system so that future contact with the allergens does not yield a dramatic response. This is the best way for a veterinarian to cure their patients' allergies.

Food allergies can also be a problem for dogs and cats. There is no definitive testing for food allergies. Instead, the veterinary dermatologist will make recommendations for foods that are a novel protein or a hydrolyzed protein. This diet is fed over six to eight weeks, and the dermatologist will monitor the response to the food. While waiting for this food trial to yield results, dermatologists can prescribe topical and oral treatments to provide itch relief and improve the skin's ability to act as a protective barrier.

Veterinary dermatologists are also good at treating stubborn, non-healing wounds. For animals of all species, especially horses, bacterial infections can penetrate deep into the skin. They can also be complicated by bacteria that is resistant to a lot of the antibiotics that we have available today. With persistent treatments and a lot of time and patience, veterinary dermatologists can provide better comfort for their itchy patients.

Oncology

Just like humans, animals can develop different kinds of cancers. Cancer is when a cell's reproduction goes out of control and spreads into the surrounding tissues. Healthy cells in the body are trained to seek out and destroy abnormal cells and cancer cells, but when there are too many of these abnormal cells, the cancer can stick around and develop in the form of a distinct tumor. If cells of the immune system or bone marrow are involved, the cancer can be very far-reaching. Some cancers can be benign like small skin growths, but malignant cancers are the kind that can spread to other internal organs. Not all cancers can be treated in the same way.

Chemotherapy is one form of treatment that involves the use of medications to kill fast-growing cells in an animal's body. Chemotherapeutic agents come in different forms, from oral tablets to injectable medications that can only be handled by your veterinarian or veterinary oncologist. This is because chemotherapeutic drugs can be absorbed by contact. In fact, animals who have received chemotherapy will excrete it through their bodily fluids for 24 to 48 hours. This means that you should avoid contact with these fluids. Otherwise, you may absorb the drugs yourself and become very sick.

Radiation is another form of cancer treatment. It is performed at a specialty facility and involves the use of a powerful beam of energy that is focused onto a specific location in the animal's body. The radiation will kill the cancer cells, and because the radiation can be fine-tuned to a very precise region, it has a minimal impact on the healthy cells around the cancer site.

For localized tumors, especially skin tumors, surgical removal is necessary. Some general practicing vets and soft tissue surgeons may have experience with this, but surgical oncologists are specifically trained for it. It can be very tricky because certain malignant tumors (e.g. mast cell tumors) can appear small but really have a wide distribution of cancer cells in the surrounding tissues. This is why very wide and deep surgical margins are necessary to ensure that the entire tumor has been removed. If the cancer cells are left behind, the cancer will come back again. Some situations, like this one, may call for the use of other treatments like chemotherapy and radiation.

Researchers are working on the creation of vaccines as a way to combat cancer. This type of treatment is called immunotherapy. Like regular vaccines, these special vaccines have small amounts of DNA from the cancer cells that the immune system will use to recognize and destroy diseased cells in the future. For example, there are melanoma vaccines available for dogs and horses. Melanoma is a type of cancer that occurs on the skin, around the eyes, and sometimes in the mouth. When an animal is diagnosed, the vaccine can be used to help train the immune system to seek out and destroy any recurring melanoma in the body. Studies show they are very effective.

If these types of treatments are not an option for a cancer patient, oncologists can also help with palliative therapy and pain management. Palliative therapy is a type of treatment that is meant to help reduce the pain and suffering that comes from dealing with a severe illness like cancer. Oral and sometimes topical medications can help relieve pain. Acupuncture, supplements, and chiropractic work can also help.

Ophthalmology

Ophthalmology is the study of the eye and its associated disorders. Even though animals don't wear eyeglasses, they might need to have their eyes examined regularly, especially if there is a problem. Most general practicing vets are able to perform basic eye testing. They can check the pressure inside of the eye, and they can make sure there isn't an issue like dry eye or a scratch on the eye (called a corneal ulcer).

Animals can develop some of the same eye problems that humans can. For example, they can develop cataracts, which are opacities that affect the clear disc inside of the eye called the lens. The lens focuses light onto the back of the eye so that vision can be processed. When the fibers inside of the lens become diseased, it obscures the passage of light so that vision cannot be processed normally. Cataracts can occur due to old age or due to other diseases like diabetes mellitus. Veterinary ophthalmologists can perform surgery on small and large animals by removing the diseased lens and replacing it with an artificial one.

Glaucoma is the disease that occurs when there is increased pressure inside the eye. There are different structures in the eye that produce a fluid called aqueous humor which supplies nutrients to the inner eye structures. This fluid is created by the ciliary body and drained through the iridocorneal angle. When there is a problem with the iridocorneal angle, and fluid cannot drain effectively, the fluid has nowhere to go.

This causes an increase in pressure. The veterinary ophthalmologist can prescribe medications to help with this problem, but in some cases, eye surgery may be necessary.

Animals can also develop diseases affecting their eyelids. Eyelids that roll inward too far (entropion) and eyelids that roll outward too far (ectropion) can be surgically corrected by veterinarians. Sometimes, small cysts or tumors can grow on the eyelids, and surgery is necessary to remove them. In trauma cases with small dogs or dogs with shallow eye sockets, the eyeball can pop out and become trapped by the eyelids. A procedure called a tarsorrhaphy involves pushing the eyeball back into place and then surgically closing the eyelids. The sutures that close the eyelids are removed after 10-14 days.

There are lots of topical medications that ophthalmologists can prescribe. Animals with glaucoma or dry eye can be kept comfortable with different ointments or drops. If the condition does not respond to medications, or the patient is in a lot of pain, surgical removal of the eye may be recommended.

Emergency and critical care

Most veterinarians work during the daytime hours and see patients by appointment. The occasional emergency may occur during the daytime, and some general practicing vets are able to accommodate these patients as work-ins. But just like in human medicine, true emergencies or overnight emergencies need to go to an emergency hospital. This is especially the case if the daytime veterinarian does not offer overnight emergency services.

All emergency patients are triaged. This means that they are evaluated by veterinary staff to determine their level of urgency. The most urgent patients are the ones that are losing a lot of blood, are having trouble breathing, have collapsed, or are unconscious. Vomiting, diarrhea, injury, and pain are also reasons that an animal will need to go to the emergency room. If a patient needs continuous hospital care with various treatments or intravenous fluids, they might transfer to an emergency vet overnight and then go back to their regular vet the following day.

Emergency veterinarians are trained to perform life-saving procedures. They can perform emergency surgeries like when a dog develops a condition known as gastric dilatation volvulus (GDV). Also known as "bloat," this is when a dog's stomach becomes very distended due to gas or food, and then it flips over on itself. GDV can be fatal without immediate surgery and intensive aftercare. In horses, colic can occur. This is a generalized term for when horses have a problem with their gastrointestinal tract. If there is an obstruction, surgery must be performed to relieve it.

Emergency vets can help with other critical patients. If a dog or cat presents with acute respiratory distress, this means they are having trouble breathing. Certain lung diseases or issues with the heart can cause pets to have trouble breathing. These patients are placed inside of an oxygen cage and are given medications so that they can breathe better. If there is fluid around the lungs, the fluid can be removed so that the patient can breathe better while the fluid is tested to look for a cause of illness. If a patient is in distress because they have lost a lot of blood, emergency vets can start giving a blood transfusion.

Internal medicine

Also known as internists, internal medicine specialists will see patients with more complicated medical histories. By applying additional training and scientific knowledge of the internal organs to clinical experience, internists can help patients with almost any disease or multiple diseases. They also have the tools to perform diagnostics that would otherwise be invasive or unable to be performed by a general practicing veterinarian. Internists will see a wide variety of cases, some of which may fall under different scientific categories such as theriogenology, the study of reproductive medicine.

There are a number of infectious diseases that can cause illness in animals. Many will present with fever, lethargy, and anorexia, but it can be difficult to determine where the infection is coming from. Some patients are diagnosed with a fever of unknown origin. Internists are skilled at creating a problem list, which is a list of all the possible causes of the patient's infection. Diagnostics such as blood work, urine testing, x-rays, culture and sensitivity testing, and blood cultures can help narrow the list down. If an airway infection is suspected, internists can collect fluid and cell samples from the airways to rule out a bacterial infection versus a viral or fungal infection.

Endocrinology is the study of diseases that are caused by hormones. Diseases like hypothyroidism (an underactive thyroid gland), Cushing's disease (an overactive adrenal gland), and diabetes mellitus (insufficient insulin or lack of a response to insulin in the body) are all problems that fall under the endocrine disease category. Endocrine diseases can be difficult to manage, and sometimes it seems like no two patients are alike! For example, diabetes in dogs is typically treated with diet change and insulin injections. Insulin is the hormone produced by the pancreas and allows sugar from food to be taken up by cells for an energy source. It takes close monitoring and repeat testing to figure out how much insulin will be needed for a diabetic patient. This process can take several weeks, and then blood levels need to be monitored every three to six months or any time that a diabetic patient is ill.

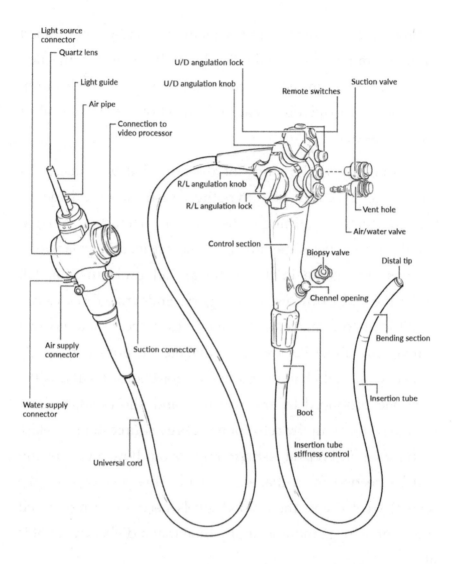

Light source connector
Quartz lens
U/D angulation lock
Light guide
U/D angulation knob
Suction valve
Remote switches
Air pipe
Connection to video processor
R/L angulation knob
R/L angulation lock
Vent hole
Air/water valve
Control section
Biopsy valve
Distal tip
Channel opening
Bending section
Air supply connector
Suction connector
Insertion tube
Water supply connector
Boot
Insertion tube stiffness control
Universal cord

Internists can also work with tools that a general practicing vet might not have. Endoscopy is a type of procedure that is considered to be non-invasive. It involves the use of a camera and light on the end of a long tube. This tube is placed into the trachea (aka windpipe) in order to evaluate the small airways that lead into the lungs. Alternatively, the endoscope can be placed down through the esophagus and into the stomach. It can also be placed into the colon through the rectum, which is a procedure called a colonoscopy. In any of these situations, the internist can look for evidence of inflammation or disease. Sometimes, parasitic worms can be visualized, or a tumor or polyp may be discovered. Fluid samples and small tissue samples can be collected through a special port in the endoscope tube. Most patients who undergo endoscopic procedures, especially small animals, are under general anesthesia.

Anesthesiology

Veterinary anesthesiologists specialize in the monitoring of patients while they are sedated or unconscious for surgical and dental procedures. They also prescribe medications to relieve pain during and after these procedures. In specialty hospitals, there is usually a dedicated anesthesiologist to focus on the patient's vital signs and state of consciousness while the specialty surgeon or dentist focuses on the patient's procedure.

Anesthesiologists utilize monitoring equipment that is identical to what is used in human anesthesiology. Machines are used to monitor heart rate, blood pressure, and the saturation of oxygen in a patient's blood. Anesthesiologists are also in charge of picking the right kind of intravenous fluids that are used to support a patient undergoing surgery. They can also administer medications for certain situations. For example, if a patient's blood pressure starts to decrease, anesthesiologists can make adjustments to fluid rate and the rate of anesthetic gas being delivered. If this doesn't help, a medication can be given intravenously to help increase blood pressure. Anesthesiologists can also intervene when emergencies happen, like if a patient's heart were to stop beating.

Pain management is also a big part of an anesthesiologist's job. Intensive surgeries like orthopedic procedures can be extremely painful. These patients will need much stronger and longer-lasting pain medications compared to a patient who has undergone a minor procedure. Pain medications can be injectable ones that are delivered in small doses constantly, or they can be oral or topical medications that are given at scheduled times when a patient is recovering from surgery.

Radiology

Radiology is when imaging devices are utilized to diagnose a patient. Veterinarians use the same imaging modalities that human doctors use. X-rays or radiographs are the most commonly used images, and they are carried by many general practice hospitals. Doctors will use x-rays to look for broken bones, intestinal obstructions or foreign bodies, bladder stones, enlarged or shrunken internal organs, bloat or GDV, arthritis, heart disease, lung disease, and certain types of cancer. Veterinarians can specialize in the study of radiology and generate reports based on images that are submitted for review. This is a great service because there are so many little details that the average vet might miss on initial x-ray interpretation.

Boarded veterinary radiologists are also trained to use ultrasound equipment. Ultrasound is when a high-frequency sound wave is used to create an image. When an ultrasound test is performed, doctors can see inside internal organs whereas x-rays may have some limitations, but that's not to say that x-rays don't have some benefit over ultrasound. Every situation is different, but lots of information can be gathered from these imaging modalities.

There are some situations where small and large animals need to have CT or MRI scans. These are large machines that can provide detailed imaging of trickier areas like inside the nasal cavity, the skull, and around the spinal cord. These images are especially useful for surgical planning and for oncologists who are trying to determine how deep a tumor attaches into surrounding tissues. Animal patients may only need mild sedation for x-rays and ultrasound, but CT and MRI patients need to be completely still. This means that general anesthesia is necessary.

Pathology

The study of the cause and effects of disease in animals is called pathology. Pathologists provide an abundance of information to other veterinarians. Clinical pathologists are the doctors who look at blood samples for evidence of disease, look at cells collected from a tumor to see what type it is, and run numerous other diagnostics involving the use of tissue samples from patients. When specialized tests are necessary for their patients, general practicing vets might collect samples and submit them to reference laboratories where boarded pathologists can help run tests.

Anatomic pathologists are the veterinarians that study patients who are deceased. When a human pathologist examines the body of another human, this is called an autopsy. When a veterinary pathologist examines the body of an animal, it is called a necropsy. Necropsies can provide a lot of information besides just the cause of death for a patient. For example, if a very young puppy dies suddenly, a necropsy would be useful to make sure that the other puppies in the litter will be okay. Anatomic pathologists can also submit testing for patients who were tentatively diagnosed with rabies.

Integrative medicine

Much of what we know about veterinary medicine is derived from scientific studies and clinical data, and this is sometimes referred to as Western medicine. Holistic medicine involves Eastern medicine practices like acupuncture and the use of herbal supplements. Integrative medicine combines elements of both Western and Eastern medicine in order to find the best ways to treat a patient. This has its benefits when other treatment options have been exhausted, and it may also minimize some of the side effects that patients experience with traditional medications.

Acupuncture is the practice of using very thin needles and inserting them into certain points on the body. By doing this, they can alter the flow of energy called qi (or "chi") along a track of points referred to as a meridian. You can think of a meridian as a string of pearls linking these points together, and there are multiple meridians that cover different body parts. When an animal has an illness or medical problem, acupuncturists work to determine the cause by deciding if there is a qi deficiency (low energy flow) or qi stagnation (no energy flow, or an obstruction to flow). By placing acupuncture needles in strategic locations, acupuncturists can improve the flow of energy, which helps to correct the medical problem. Acupuncture can be used for a wide array of health problems such as arthritis pain, inflammation, skin issues, and behavioral disorders.

Herbal supplements are also a part of integrative medicine and what is called traditional Chinese veterinary medicine (TCVM). All medications that humans and animals take contain active ingredients, some of which are derived from plants and herbs. In herbal medicine, the original plant or plant extract is utilized for treatments. There are many herbal supplements, so it is important to have an accurate diagnosis from a veterinary herbalist before picking a supplement. One of the most commonly used herbal supplements is yunnan baiyao. It is known for its wound healing properties and its ability to help stop bleeding. Vets will prescribe it for dogs who have bleeding problems or who have certain types of cancer like splenic hemangiosarcoma.

Physical therapy and rehabilitation are elements that are commonly incorporated into integrative medical treatments. Sports injuries, musculoskeletal injuries, post-surgery recovery, and arthritis are the most common issues where physical therapy can improve healing time and minimize discomfort. Physical therapy involves passive range of motion exercises, which involve the movement of a limb while the patient is not bearing weight on it. The limb may be extended and flexed repetitively, in slow movements, and deep tissue massage can help with inflammation by improving blood flow. Swim therapy is another part of physical therapy because it helps patients to move their bodies yet greatly decreases the strain from the patient's body weight. Cold laser therapy, which involves the use of a low energy beam of light, can be used to improve blood flow to a targeted area and can help with wound healing.

Nutrition is another element of integrative medicine. This is because holistic medicine and integrative medicine involve a "whole animal" approach to diagnosis and treatment. Thus it is important to think about what an animal is eating! Veterinary nutritionists are experts who know all of the essential nutrients that a patient will need. This is especially important in an age where there are too many commercial diets available, and consumers might select the wrong diet for their pet. For example, some dog owners feel that home-cooked meals might be better than commercial diets, but commercial diets are guaranteed to have the right balance of a dog's essential nutrients. Simply feeding your dog cooked chicken and rice and broccoli is not a balanced diet, and it can lead to health problems.

Large animal medicine

Just like small animal medicine, there are general practicing and specialty large animal veterinarians. They can do many of the same things small animal vets can, but the work environment can be *very* different! Most large animal vets travel great distances to see their patients. They may drive to an owner's barn in order to examine a horse, or they might have to rope an injured calf in the field and repair the wound right there. Specialty hospitals mostly operate out of large buildings that have wide hallways, large stalls for hospitalized patients, and large operating rooms for surgical patients. Some of the above-mentioned specialties may focus on small animal species versus large animals, but others like ophthalmologists, cardiologists, and anesthesiologists often work with small *and* large animals.

Food animal medicine

This area is a little different from large animal medicine because it focuses on the care of animals involved in food production. Some of the same rules apply between food animals and large animals, but the majority of the work is done outdoors on farms. Cattle, pigs, chickens, and sheep are some of the animals that food animal vets work with, but it isn't just about meat production. Eggs, milk, wool, and fiber products also fall into this category.

Food animal vets must ensure that farm animals are healthy. They routinely visit these locations to provide vaccines for healthy animals and to provide medications and treatments for sick animals. These vets must be careful when prescribing medications because certain antibiotics, for example, can remain in the muscles or milk of cattle. The use of these antibiotics is illegal because of the potential harm if the product is consumed by humans.

Reproductive medicine is an important part of food animal medicine. It is the vet's job to ensure that healthy babies are born. They can also travel to farms and use ultrasound equipment to determine if an animal is pregnant. If there are birthing difficulties, food animal vets are trained to assist. These can be emergency situations, in which case large animal emergency veterinarians can be contacted.

Zoo animals and wildlife

Zoo animal medicine is the most diverse field because the care and treatment of every other species of animal falls into this category. Some small animal vets who focus on dogs and cats may have expertise or experience in treating "pocket pets" like rodents and guinea pigs, or reptiles, birds, and fish. These small animal vets will sometimes be referred to as exotic veterinarians, and they might see all of these patients under one roof. Zoo medicine also has boarded specialists who have completed an internship and residency after veterinary school. These specialists may work in veterinary schools, in zoos, or literally out in the field because it can be difficult to walk a giraffe or an elephant into a building if the hospital isn't big enough. Veterinarians who work with animals that are not owned by people or zoos are also called wildlife veterinarians.

Many veterinary schools have teaching hospitals, which are functioning hospitals with veterinarians and veterinary students. The hospitals are broken up into different departments, some of which involve the care of species besides dogs, cats, and horses. The zoo medicine department at my vet school (the University of Florida) was *always* busy, and there were so many interesting patients! We had resident gopher tortoises who were being rehabilitated for future re-release, and we also had resident tarantulas. During appointments, we would see anything from large parrots owned by clients to owls that belonged to zoos and wildlife sanctuaries. We helped squirrels and various small rodents. On occasion, we helped with diagnostic imaging for alligators and tigers!

As a student, I was also able to help on field trips to zoos. The veterinarians in charge of examining and treating the patients had a list of animals to see for the day. One by one, each patient would be brought into the room by a zookeeper. We started by helping a hedgehog with an oral tumor and ended with a two-year-old male puma who was being seen for his annual physical exam. The veterinarian in charge had to ensure that the puma was tranquilized for his examination so that he would not become too stressed, although it was a little scary riding in the van next to him on our way back to his enclosure, knowing he could start moving around again at any moment.

Tranquilization is one of the ways that vets can help manage stressed animals, especially wildlife and those animals who would otherwise not have exposure to humans. Many of the wild animals who need veterinary care are already stressed because they are injured or in need of rescuing from a dangerous situation. Smaller animals may be a little easier to handle, but how does one go about helping an injured deer or elk if the patient keeps running away? Wildlife vets receive special training for the use of dart guns and blow darts. These are special needles that can be propelled toward an animal, and when the needle connects, it injects sedatives or tranquilizers to help the animal relax and lie down on the ground. If there is a wound, a wildlife vet can help treat the wound there in the field. In serious cases, transport may need to be arranged to get the sick animal to a hospital.

Aquatic medicine

Similar to zoo medicine, aquatic vets handle many different species that vary from the very small to the *very* large! These animals spend almost all of their time in the water, so aquatic vets will help dolphins, turtles, whales, otters, sea lions, crabs, octopus, penguins, and even jellyfish! Some aquatic vets might oversee the care of fish in an aquaculture setting (think like agriculture, but instead of plants, fish are cultivated). Other aquatic vets will help to care for animals in zoos, aquariums, and other locations like Sea World. They can also help with wildlife and are an important part of conservation and research programs, offering valuable information such as the effects of climate change on aquatic animal and coral reef populations.

Many of the ways that general practicing vets treat their patients can be applied to aquatic animals, especially marine mammals. Certain medications, surgeries, and treatments can be given or modified to make it more appropriate for aquatic patients. For other species, like fish, aquatic vets have different methods. Fish can develop tumors just like dogs and cats can. Certain tumors can be surgically removed, but the patient should be under general anesthesia when this happens so that he is free of stress and pain. A special anesthetic drug is put into the fish's water so that he becomes unconscious, and because fish constantly need water flowing over their gills to help them stay oxygenated, a tube is placed in the fish's mouth which forces anesthesia-infused water through the gills. This way, the fish is asleep and not feeling any pain while surgery occurs.

Shelter medicine

Some veterinarians work directly with homeless animals or with pets who require low-cost veterinary care. This is where shelter veterinarians can help. These are the vets who work in animal shelters or humane societies. They ensure that animals are healthy before they can be adopted. Shelter vets ensure that animals are vaccinated and have been spayed or neutered, thus having a significant impact on the reduction of pet overpopulation. It is estimated that millions of unwanted animals are euthanized in shelters every year in the United States.

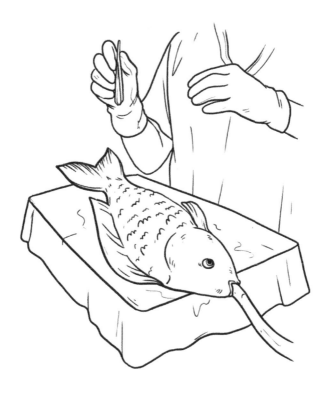

Spay and neuter surgeries involve the removal of specific reproductive organs so that pets cannot have babies. Shelter veterinarians have lots of experience with these surgeries, and many of their patients heal quickly! Shelter vets will also examine each new animal who comes into the shelter, making sure they are free from disease.

Abandoned animals are also brought to the shelter, and if the animals are injured or in pain, shelter vets will provide the care that they need. In the event of animal cruelty or neglect, local authorities and the county's animal control service may ask shelter vets to examine the animal and offer expert opinions about that animal's health.

Most animal shelters focus on the care of dogs and cats, but some will see exotics like rabbits and guinea pigs. Some shelter vets are also trained to help with large animals like horses and goats. In some situations, shelters may offer low-cost clinics so that families with financial difficulties can bring their pets for an examination, vaccinations, and medical treatments.

Lab animal medicine

Veterinarians can also specialize in working with the animals that are used in research studies. These vets are called laboratory animal veterinarians. They ensure the proper care of research animals while also helping with the collection of data for research purposes. Rodents like mice and rats are the most common species included in medical studies because their biology is so similar to our own. We both age in the same ways, but the rat's life cycle is shorter, making him an ideal research model because it would take decades to study the same things in humans. Lab animal vets also work with larger species like primates, pigs, and sheep. Each day, veterinarians will examine these research animals to ensure that they are happy and free from disease and pain. In the event that a lab animal is suffering, the lab animal vet ensures that the animal can pass peacefully.

Education and teaching

Some veterinarians choose to stay in academia when they've graduated. Even some of the vets who've chosen to go into private practice may one day decide to teach veterinary students. Not only is this a great way to learn new information about veterinary medicine, it is also a fun way to help guide new veterinarians. Almost all of the veterinarians who choose to do an internship or residency after veterinary school will teach to some degree. This is because lectures and case rounds are requirements for these positions. If a specialty veterinarian chooses to work at the hospital of a veterinary school, the same criteria apply. In fact, many of these vets are the professors who teach students in vet school.

These teaching veterinarians will provide lectures in a classroom setting, and they will create the quizzes and tests necessary to pass the class. Some of these teaching vets will work with students directly on the clinic floor. They oversee the caseloads for the vet students and ensure that medical records are accurate. You might also find veterinarians teaching classes at schools for veterinary technicians and at continuing education (CE) events. In order to keep a doctor's license in good standing with the veterinary board and the state in which the doctor practices, a certain number of hours of continuing education are required every two years. This consists of live or pre-recorded lectures on almost any subject pertaining to veterinary medicine.

Besides teaching, veterinarians can also educate others in the form of written communication. Some of the blogs and medical articles published online have been written by veterinarians. This book is one such example because I am a full-time small animal veterinarian who enjoys writing and teaching. Veterinarians in academia will write research articles on complicated medical and surgical information, and some contribute to the content that fills our veterinary school textbooks.

There are also veterinarians who serve as representatives for pharmaceutical and food companies. Some of the companies that create the medications, vaccines, diets, and preventatives that we prescribe work with a group of veterinarians. These vets can provide feedback and can serve as representatives who visit animal hospitals and talk with other doctors. They can also talk to us about the latest and greatest in treatments and products.

Government and public health

There is a large group of veterinarians who work directly with the government and/or in the public health sector. Known as federal veterinarians, these doctors serve an important role in ensuring that products are safe for animal consumption *and* human consumption. They also study medications and products in order to determine adverse effects and risk factors. If there is a public health crisis or issues with communicable diseases, federal veterinarians are the main point of contact for state and local veterinarians for more information.

In the United States, some of these vets work for the United States Department of Agriculture (USDA). They can ensure the health and safety of many animals, especially farm animals, and they help establish guidelines for interstate and international travel. If you've ever needed to fly out of the country with your dog, for example, your regular veterinarian can help you determine the requirements necessary to fly. This usually involves a written health certificate that ensures your pup is healthy. Certificates are especially necessary if flying internationally, and veterinarians who work for the USDA are in charge of endorsing these certificates.

The safety and efficacy of various veterinary products and medications falls under the purview of the Food and Drug Administration (FDA). For example, in 2018, the FDA announced that it was investigating a potential link between a type of heart disease called dilated cardiomyopathy (DCM) and grain-free diets. Food companies had the idea to provide limited-ingredient diets that eliminated grain as an ingredient because it is thought to be a possible cause for allergies in dogs. However, in recent years, there has been an increase in the number of DCM cases in dogs and cats. When researchers looked for a link, grain-free diets were the common denominator. The investigation is still underway, but until its conclusion, the FDA and veterinary cardiologists warn that pet owners should be cautious when purchasing these diets.

Telemedicine

With the recent pandemic, telemedicine has become increasingly popular in human medicine. This is when a patient contacts a health professional via phone, email, text message, or video chat. The health care provider can diagnose and prescribe treatments to the patient in some cases, or they can help people determine if their medical issue is an emergency.

Some aspects of telemedicine also have their place in veterinary medicine. Veterinarians can also offer general medical advice to their clients, but in most states, it is illegal to diagnose a patient and prescribe treatment without having a valid veterinarian-client-patient-relationship (VCPR). This involves the vet having physically examined the patient in person within the span of one year. Since the pandemic, the rules have been relaxed a little, and patients with valid VCPRs are able to take advantage of telemedicine.

CHAPTER 5:

WHAT KIND OF EDUCATION IS NECESSARY BEFORE APPLYING TO VET SCHOOL?

Every prospective veterinary student must meet the same requirements and prerequisites before applying to veterinary school, but how you go about achieving these may be entirely different than others. The average veterinary student is a high school graduate who goes on to complete prerequisite courses at a four-year university and might pick up a degree or two along the way. However, I have met some veterinarians with much more interesting beginnings. In my graduating class in vet school, there was a retired commercial airline pilot, and another student had been a lawyer for several years before he decided to apply to vet school.

If you're like me and you decided on becoming a veterinarian while you were in middle school or high school, you might end up on a track that is similar to mine. I was a senior in high school when the guidance counselor asked if I had any aspirations toward a certain career. Most veterinarians will tell you that they knew they wanted to be vets since they were toddlers. I was a little late to the game, and I decided that I wanted to be a vet when I told the guidance counselor that I liked animals and I liked medicine. She told me, "You should consider veterinary school."

"Okay." And that was it. How strange is it that one short conversation with that counselor changed the entire trajectory of my life? I began to ask about the requirements for applying and where the nearest veterinary school was located. I was a student at a high school in southwest Florida, and I then learned that the only vet school in the state was the University of Florida located in north central Florida. I had never heard of it because I had only been in Florida for two years up until that point (I was born and raised in New York City). It turned out that the University of Florida was and still is one of the top veterinary schools in the country, and it provided me with an excellent education that will help me for years to come.

There are only 28 accredited veterinary schools in the United States, and the competition is always high when it comes to quality of the applicants. It is estimated that only 10 to 15 percent of people who apply to veterinary school will be accepted. Some students are accepted on their first try while others might apply a second or third or even a fourth time. One of my classmates applied four times before she was accepted and is now one of the best oncologists around. Veterinary schools are looking for prospective students with excellent grades, a good work ethic, extracurricular activities, and diverse backgrounds.

When applying to vet school, it helps to have a grade point average (or GPA) that's very high. Your school likely keeps track of this for you already. By taking higher difficulty classes like honors or advanced placement courses, you can get extra grade points for your GPA. Advanced placement courses can also get you on a faster track to vet school because they count for credit toward your college education.

There are some veterinary schools that only require an education level as advanced as a high school diploma. This mostly applies to some international veterinary schools because the majority of vet schools in the United States require some college or a bachelor's degree, which typically takes four years to achieve. You will choose a major for your degree, which means that out of all of your courses, most of them will track a certain specialty or field of study. In college, I majored in animal sciences or animal biology. This is a common track for veterinary students because it covers the majority of the prerequisites that you will need before applying to vet school. However, veterinary schools love students with different backgrounds, so don't be afraid of majoring in something that you are passionate about. There was a student who majored in music in my class, and he is a talented small animal veterinarian today.

Many of the prerequisites required by veterinary schools focus on math and science. These are your most important subjects because you will deal with them every day of your veterinary career. You will need to have a basic understanding of chemistry and biochemistry in order to understand how medications work, how vitamins are essential to healthy patients, and how proteins and certain elements can help move fluids and nutrients through the body. Microbiology, which is the study of microscopic organisms, is critical to our understanding of infectious diseases and how they can spread. Physics is also a requirement for many schools because it helps doctors to learn about things like heat transfer (think about patients with fevers) and fluid dynamics, like when patients develop edema due to certain health issues.

Back when I was a student, calculus was a requirement for vet school. Calculus is the study of rates of change, and it can be very complicated to understand. Most schools require it because it demonstrates that the veterinary student has a firm grasp of difficult concepts and tricky math, but in all honesty, calculus-level math does not factor into too much of my day. Algebra, however, is used daily. Doctors use algebra to calculate the dose of medications for a patient based on their weight in pounds or kilograms. It is also used to calculate the rate of fluids necessary to rehydrate a sick patient.

Statistics is the process of analyzing numerical data. If you've ever read through a clinical trial or study, you may have seen different numbers in the results section that discuss whether or not a study proved its hypothesis or had a successful response to a treatment. Doctors will look at these data to determine if the results of a study were statistically significant, meaning that the results were not an accident. So if the response to a treatment was proven to be statistically significant, it means the treatment was effective.

Veterinary schools like the University of Florida also require some advanced courses that can be more challenging, further proof that their prospective veterinary students can handle a rigorous curriculum. Animal sciences and animal nutrition were two requirements when I was a student, and they are still available to this day. I remember being excited on my first day of these classes because they were my very first courses at UF, and they were my first animal classes *ever*! My only prior experience had been firsthand with the many species of animals that I'd owned. Growing up, I had guinea pigs, hamsters, rabbits, fish, dogs, and cats. Maybe that's why it was so surprising to suddenly be listening to lectures about horses and cattle and sheep.

The rest of your prerequisites will be comprised of English classes, humanities, and social studies. Written and verbal communication are extremely important for doctors. As veterinarians, we need to take complicated medical jargon and simplify it for the general public. College-level English courses will enhance your reading comprehension and writing skills, which are important for when you are creating medical notes for your patients. Most vet schools allow a lot of freedom when it comes to the humanities and social studies courses. I remember that human psychology and physiology courses were helpful to me because some aspects of those classes could be applied to veterinary medicine. I also took astronomy and history courses just because I love those subjects so much, and they did help in that they were research-heavy and writing-intensive courses.

Some students may choose to start their college courses early by taking advanced placement classes. I did not because I had moved states twice in my high school years. In each high school that I attended, teachers noticed my grades and skills, and they would move me to upper division classes. But with each jump to a new state, the process would start over again, so I just stayed with honors courses. Once I graduated high school, I chose to go to a two-year state college so that I could be close to my family and my high school sweetheart (now husband). State college was also a lot cheaper than a four-year university, and I could still take some of my vet school prerequisites because some veterinary schools will accept a transfer of credits. However, you should check your vet school's requirements because they may not allow certain courses at lower division levels, or they may have limits on the number of credits you can transfer. I learned this the hard way when I took a third year at my state college, and when I got into UF undergraduate to complete my four-year degree, they dropped 17 of my credit hours, including microbiology. This ended up turning my four-year degree into a five-year degree, but I didn't mind because my time at UF as an undergraduate was so fun and exciting!

Most veterinary schools prefer that you take your prerequisites at a four-year college because the work may be a bit more challenging, further proof that you are an excellent vet school candidate. I was happy that most of my credits transferred, but now I had to take microbiology again. This time, I found the information extremely complicated. The subject matter was not just playing with gel agar plates in a lab setting. It was also learning about semi-permeable membranes of cells and how lots of little letters that signify the chemical elements will interact with channels across the membranes to allow passage in and out of cells. I had *such* a hard time trying to retain this information, and my first couple of exams were almost failing. I decided to get with a friend and fellow classmate who was also having a hard time with microbiology. We made a point of borrowing one of the campus study rooms for a couple of hours a week. We'd pick a private room, make sure we had our coffee handy, and we'd discuss our notes. Our grades significantly improved after that.

Many graduate schools require that you take a special test called the Graduate Record Examination or GRE. This standardized exam is very similar to the Scholastic Aptitude Test (SAT) and the American College Test (ACT) that are necessary to get into college. College students take the GRE before applying to graduate or professional schools like vet school. It analyzes your reasoning, writing, mathematical, and critical thinking skills. At the time, I remember what a grueling experience it was. A certain benchmark score is necessary for most vet schools, but if you do not meet this score requirement, you can always retake the exam. Some schools and companies also offer classes and tutors to help students with GRE test preparedness, and there are books available that provide lots of practice questions.

CHAPTER 6:

WHAT KIND OF EXPERIENCE IS NECESSARY BEFORE APPLYING?

Vet schools will look at more than just your smarts. Veterinarians must be compassionate and caring individuals, and many vet schools prefer to accept well-rounded and experienced individuals rather than just someone with the best GPA and test scores.

While it isn't necessarily a prerequisite, having prior experience at a veterinary hospital is extremely helpful in vet school. When I was a vet student, we spent our first two years in a classroom setting. At UF, the clinical year doesn't start until the summer of your second year, heading into your third year. Our first soft tissue surgery was scheduled for the spring semester of second year, and we would be working on spaying and neutering patients that would go on to be adopted through the local animal shelter. We were all prepped and ready to go on the day of surgery, and everyone had studied what they needed to, but then the instructors said, "Okay, get your patients ready." These patients needed to have their anesthesia prepped and intravenous catheters put into their arms. In my group, no one else had prior experience doing these things except for me. I had been (and still was) a veterinary technician as a part-time job, so I already knew how to measure patients for their endotracheal tubes and how to place an intravenous catheter. I made sure to talk with my job so my groupmates could have some more one-on-one experience with dogs and cats in these matters.

It can be difficult to get a job as a veterinary technician without licensing in some states. In fact, Florida is one of the few states left that allows hospitals to hire non-licensed individuals as veterinary technicians. When I was a year or two into my undergraduate career, I went looking for animal hospital experience. I was hired by a local animal hospital as a kennel technician. These are the individuals who take care of patients that are boarding at the hospital. Not every hospital has a boarding facility on site, but some do. When I wasn't walking and feeding and medicating boarders, I was in the busiest part of the hospital assisting the vet techs and doctors. I was both fascinated and terrified by the pace of the average workday, but I knew I wanted to go further.

About a year later, I made the move to Gainesville so that I could attend UF to finish my undergraduate career. I had applied to be a vet tech at several hospitals in the area, not just for the experience but also because living with my boyfriend (now husband) in another city was expensive. I was so fortunate that the practice manager of a corporate-run animal hospital was hiring. She took a chance on me, a newbie with only a year's worth of kennel experience. The techs at that hospital, two of whom would also go on to attend UF's vet school, took me under their wing and trained me. That experience was so valuable because it really helped me as a doctor. I had a better understanding of general small animal practice and had more skills than some of my classmates by the time I was in vet school. To this day, there are still some vets who struggle with the tasks that some vet techs make to look easy. I have a tremendous amount of respect and appreciation for the vet techs with whom I work, and I could not do my job if not for them.

If you are unable to obtain a job as a vet tech, or if hospitals can only hire certified veterinary technicians or CVTs, you have a few options for enhancing your work experience. Some hospitals may be willing to hire you as a non-licensed assistant. You will still get hands-on experience in a hospital setting, but you may have fewer responsibilities, and there may be some limitations with respect to treatments. If an animal hospital does not hire these kinds of assistants, you can ask if they would accept any volunteers. Most hospitals can do this as long as you are older than 18, possibly 16 in some states. Animal shelters can especially benefit from volunteers, and you would also be doing a great service for your community.

Extracurricular activities are a plus when it comes to applying to vet school. The average veterinarian doesn't just eat, sleep, and breathe veterinary medicine. It is better to show that you have other interests outside of vet med. It shows that you have a good work-life balance, which is a critical skill in this fast-paced field because it helps you maintain good physical and mental health. Some extracurriculars consist of school clubs, sports, and other activities. These can be pertinent to veterinary medicine, but it is completely okay if they aren't. In my case, I decided that I wanted to take up dance again in college. I was active in ballet and gymnastics when I was much younger, and a local dance studio offered ballet classes for adults. It was a great way to exercise each week, and I *loved* being able to dance again.

Most vet schools in the United States only accept applications once a year, while some international schools may take applications two or three times a year. When you apply, you will likely use the VMCAS database. VMCAS stands for Veterinary Medical College Application Service. This way, if you decide to apply to multiple vet schools, which may slightly increase your chances of acceptance, you will only have to fill out the one application. Because of my family and my husband's family, I decided against applying out of state and only applied to UF. Some schools may have you fill out an additional application that is solely for the one school. Many schools require an entrance essay that details why you want to go to vet school or why you might be a great fit. It can be so difficult to write an original essay that stands out from the thousands of others!

When applying, you will also need some letters of recommendation. The people who write these letters should be people that you've worked with or people that know you best. Most vet schools prefer that you do not ask your parents as they will probably be a little biased about why you are the most amazing candidate. I asked one of the vets at my job to write a letter for me. I also asked my tech manager, our practice manager, and one of my teachers to write letters for me. The letters will explain why you are a good fit for vet school and what you bring to the table that stands out from other perspective students.

CHAPTER 7:

WHAT ARE THE NEXT STEPS AFTER YOU APPLY?

Waiting is probably the worst part of all! Most vet school applications are due by end of summer or beginning of fall. It takes a lot of time for the admissions board to go through those hundreds, if not thousands, of applications. This usually means that you will receive a letter a little bit before or by the beginning of the new year.

Your letter might say that you've been granted an interview. This means that you will go to the veterinary school and sit before a group of people who are part of the school's admissions board. They will ask you lots of different questions, but some of them are repeated each year. This might give you the chance to think about how you'd like to answer. Sample questions include:

- Why do you want to go to veterinary school?
- How do you stand out from other applicants?
- Why did you specifically apply to this school's program?

- Have you ever been in a situation where you disagreed with someone?
- How do you feel about ethical issues (e.g. convenience euthanasia)?
- How do you plan to finance your vet school education?

Your interviewers may also ask a "what would you do" type question, like how you would approach a colleague who was doing something wrong in school or at work. They are curious to know more about you, what makes you different, and how you will function in a busy and often stressful role. Keep in mind that there really aren't any right or wrong answers here. Your interviewers' main goal is to see that you are clear in your answers, that you can explain yourself well, and that you can answer quickly without delaying or fumbling with your words. As mentioned above, communication is extremely important in veterinary medicine.

Interviewers will ask you about the cost of your education because this is a big problem in our field right now. It is *very* expensive to go to veterinary school or any medical professional school at a graduate level. Many human doctors and dentists have higher salaries than other medical professions, so it may be feasible for them to pay for their education via student loans that are to be paid back over time after they've graduated. Unfortunately, many veterinarians have a much lower income compared to other medical professions. This means that a vet's debt-to-income ratio is very high, and so it may be difficult to pay off student loans after graduation. There are income-based programs available that can help lower your monthly payments, but with higher interest rates, it can seem impossible to make even the smallest dent in the amount that you owe. When possible, you should only borrow the absolute minimum amount of money needed for college and vet school. If there are scholarships and grants, you need to apply for them because these are monies toward school that do not need to be paid back.

CHAPTER 8:

WHAT HAPPENS IF YOU DON'T GET ACCEPTED INTO VET SCHOOL?

About a month or two after the interviews, the acceptance letters are sent out to the applicants. Opening that acceptance letter can be one of the happiest days of your life! However, only 100 to 120 acceptance letters are sent out for the entire applicant pool for each school. This means that you might get a much more heartbreaking letter in the mail.

I was one of these people. On my first try applying to vet school, I didn't even receive an interview. But I took advice from some of my co-workers who said that I could contact the school for an exit interview. This is when you speak with someone in the admissions office, and they can talk to you about your application. Their advice is very valuable because they will tell you what your strongest qualities are and what are some areas where you can improve. In my case, I had good work experience and extracurriculars. My GRE score was only slightly above the benchmark requirement, and I didn't have very strong grades in some of my upper division courses. My GPA was a 3.1 while the school mostly looked for candidates closer to 3.6 and higher. This admissions counselor suggested that I prove myself by taking some upper division coursework at a graduate school level.

In 2008, the year that I graduated with my bachelor's degree, I decided to work on a certificate in public health at UF's College of Public Health and Health Professions. It was only five courses long, but it was coursework at a graduate school level and offered subjects that would be helpful for vet school. I aced all of my classes, proving that I could handle upper division coursework. During this academic year, I also continued working at my vet tech job, continued ballet classes, and tried taking the GRE again. The score didn't improve by much, but I was still happy that I survived it (again).

I applied to vet school a second time in the fall of 2008, but this time, I got an interview! I went to the vet school in February of 2009 and interviewed with three admissions board members. They asked me a lot of the interview questions discussed above, and I was so nervous that I'm certain I fumbled a response or two. That lack of confidence is probably the reason why I received a denial letter a month later. I was devastated! I spoke to the associate dean of the vet school for my exit interview. He told me that there really wasn't anything else I should change. While I was initially sad, I felt a little more confident when he told me this. Applying to vet school is so competitive, and there aren't many people along the way who will tell you that you're worth it, that you're good enough to be a veterinarian. When the associate dean told me that I was a solid candidate for vet school, it bolstered my confidence and the belief that I was good enough. I knew that I would simply try again the following year.

It was July of 2009 when my husband and I were getting situated in our bigger apartment in Gainesville, and I was contemplating more upper division work in the hopes that it would make me stand out even further in that year's applicant pool. So here I was, thinking about the class of 2014 while getting ready for work, and then I received a phone call. I didn't recognize the number, and I almost didn't answer it, but I did anyway. It was the associate dean of the vet school. "I'd like to offer you a seat in the UF College of Veterinary Medicine Class of 2013."

I didn't say anything for about ten seconds, maybe longer, because I'm certain my brain shut down and rebooted like a computer. I wasn't sure if I had heard him correctly, and my memory is a little fuzzy, but I think I said something along the lines of, "Really?" and "Do you need me to pay you now?" I didn't know if the call was intended to set up payment for tuition or not, but really, what a weird thing to say to the associate dean of your new school! I imagine other veterinary students had much more professional or eloquent responses than mine. As the associate dean continued talking to me about what a great school this was, like he was trying his hardest to convince me to accept, I was silently dancing in my living room and thinking about whom I was going to call first. I'd finally gotten into vet school!

There are lots of veterinary students with stories similar to mine. They may have been denied multiple times without even having been offered an interview. My best friend in undergraduate changed her mind about vet school for now. She is a full-time vet tech but might decide on vet school again in the future. My closest friend in vet school was originally from out of state and had been denied three times by her nearest vet school. She'd applied to UF the same year and was accepted into my class. She is now the head veterinarian at a county-run animal shelter. One of my friends from undergraduate applied to UF three times and was denied, so she applied to an out-of-state school and got accepted. She moved back to Florida after graduating. My study buddy from microbiology was worried about her grades and GPA, so she applied to an international school that had a lower benchmark requirement. She is now a successful chief of staff in North Carolina.

My acceptance into vet school wasn't quite how I'd imagined it. In a way, I had been waitlisted. This means that the school offers a number of seats to certain individuals. If any of them declines, a seat opens up, and a person on the wait list is offered the seat instead. Vet schools are increasing class sizes each year because there is a growing demand for veterinarians. This means that more seats will be available to applicants. You may choose to keep applying until you are accepted, or you might try applying out of state or internationally. In any case, your hard work and persistence will help you succeed.

CHAPTER 9:

WHAT IS VETERINARY SCHOOL LIKE?

Most veterinary schools will have a few days of freshmen orientation in the beginning. This gives you an opportunity to tour the school, get your class schedule, and get to know your fellow classmates. Some of the clubs in vet school will also be in attendance and try to recruit you if you're interested. Each school is different, and when I was a freshman, we had team-building activities at a sleepaway camp. I had never really camped before, so it was an odd experience, but it was great getting to know everyone.

At UF, there is a Big-Little program for the students. When you're a freshman, you are assigned a sophomore student to be your Big Brother or Big Sister. These sophomores usually keep a box of old notes, study guides, and quizzes that they donate to you to help you in your first year. My Big was awesome! And she gave me a huge box that became extremely helpful. She was also available to answer any questions that I had, and she remained in close contact with me throughout the rest of my vet school career. I vowed early on to be just as helpful to my Littles whenever they came along. It was a good thing I made electronic copies of all these "box" items and my notes and study guides because I would end up with *two* Little Sisters in sophomore year, so it was easier to share my things with them!

Almost all veterinary school programs are four years long. At some international schools where a four-year degree and college coursework aren't required, the vet school program is five years. At UF, the first two years are dedicated to classroom work and lab exercises. The summer between your sophomore year and junior year is when clinical rotations start, and then you're back in the classroom again in the middle of your junior year. After one more summer break, your first semester as a senior is spent in the classroom, and your spring semester has you back on the clinic floor until you graduate. In some vet schools, this setup may be different. Some schools have you focus on classroom work for the first three years, and then you spend your final year on clinical rotations.

The first year is dedicated to courses that discuss the body systems of animals with an emphasis on what is considered normal or non-diseased. I was taking three to four classes at any given time, and the classes met almost every day of the school week. The schedule was from eight in the morning to three or sometimes five in the afternoon. My initial classes included embryology, endocrinology, professional development, and anatomy. We would sit through lectures in the morning, break for lunch, and then go to the anatomy lab in the afternoon. In anatomy, we studied the structures of the dog. Each day, we would go through a different body system and identify the names of all of the body parts. Some names were much more complicated than others, like the extensor carpi radialis muscle (a band of muscle that stretches across the top of a dog's forearm).

Our anatomy class had occasional quizzes to make sure that we remembered what we learned. Because there is so much information, anatomy stretched out into the entire semester. For the other courses, however, they would only last for three to four weeks. At the end of the course, there would be one exam. Unless there were occasional homework assignments or quizzes, that one exam carried 100 percent of the weight of your grade! Some of the smaller, shorter courses were grouped into one category like small animal medicine, and so a bad grade in one of those courses could be helped with better grades in another. For the rest of the courses, a failing grade will stick, and you will need to speak with the Academic Advancement Committee. If your GPA is too low, the AAC will meet with you and determine if you will continue on with your classmates, continue with probation, or be held back a year.

Sophomore year was even more rigorous than freshman year. Classes were still taught Monday through Friday from eight in the morning to three in the afternoon, but there were many more subjects in the fall semester, so the final exams for these classes would come up much more quickly. Sometimes, there was a week with three finals in it, so all of your free time was devoted to studying. In my case, I would study late into the night before an exam just so I could cram more information into my head. I thought I was doing okay in school, but the number of courses and exams became difficult for me to balance, and I had a run-in with the Academic Advancement Committee at the end of the semester.

Looking back, I forget how low my GPA had become, but it was enough that I needed to speak with the AAC to determine if I could continue with my classmates into the following semester. It was agreed that if I could pull up my grades in the spring semester, they would let me continue. I was able to do just that! The spring semester had more classes that focused on disease in animals, but it was also our first introduction into small animal surgery. This would be the course where we veterinary students would perform our first spay and neuter surgeries.

Our surgery patients were dogs from the local animal shelter that needed to be spayed or neutered before they could be put up for adoption. In fact, many of the surgery patients for our class ended up being adopted by their surgeons. These surgeries are important because it is difficult to learn how to perform surgery by just reading about it in a textbook. Professors and other veterinarians guided us through the surgeries so that our patients would be safe. In my surgery group of three students, we were in charge of a male

Chihuahua for his neuter surgery, and the following week, we had a mixed breed terrier for her spay surgery. Both of our patients recovered very nicely and were adopted into loving homes. The experience of scrubbing in for our first surgery was scary, but in the end, we felt much more confident knowing that we were improving our surgical skills leading up to graduation in a few short years.

It is important to note that there are two different types of surgical patients in vet schools. There are patients who are woken up after their surgeries, but then there are patients who are euthanized after surgeries. The latter are referred to as terminal surgeries. Dog patients from a lab animal setting are brought in specifically for the purpose of practicing techniques like spleen removals and liver lobe removals, but then the patient is not woken up after the surgery. Terminal surgeries used to be quite commonplace among veterinary schools, but over time, many of us agreed that these are inhumane. Thus, almost all vet schools have moved away from this practice. Many schools like UF now rely on synthetic cadavers for this kind of surgical training. If you attend a vet school that still performs terminal surgeries for training purposes, you are permitted to opt out of this if you feel uncomfortable.

As the end of the spring semester of sophomore year drew closer, we were starting to get excited about two major upcoming events: coating ceremony and the start of clinical rotations. Coating ceremony is when you receive your doctor's coat, a long-sleeved white lab coat with your name embroidered on it. Some veterinary schools coat their students during freshman orientation, but UF liked to wait until right before clinical rotations. This way, the coating ceremony could mark another important achievement, which is the completion of two long years of coursework. I was so happy to have all of my family there, and I asked one of the doctors I'd worked with to be there to coat me. It was a great day!

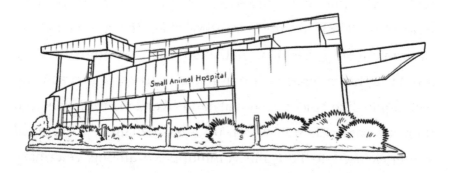

We had our clinical orientation the following week. Students in their clinical rotations are provided with firsthand experience working with the patients that are seen by vets in the small animal and large animal hospitals. These teaching hospitals work in the exact same way that other hospitals do, though the number of patients seen each day is much higher than your average private practice. In UF's case, the Small Animal Hospital is a gigantic three-story building with multiple departments. Behind it, there is an equally colossal large animal hospital for equine and other large patients. Because of having to walk back and forth between different hospitals and departments, I wore out three pairs of shoes in my first clinical year!

Over the span of a week, we were brought into the department of whichever rotation would be our first one. We shadowed the senior students who were wrapping up their clinical year *and* their entire vet school career. They taught us how to use the computer software for the vet school's small and large animal hospitals, and we learned how to manage our caseloads and type up patient notes. We also had to get used to knowing where everything was. My first rotation was internal medicine, arguably one of the most difficult rotations, so I had to know how to get to the pharmacy, radiology and ultrasound, endoscopy, and anesthesia. On that final day of orientation, the seniors left us around noon, and we were on our own.

Many of the patients who are seen by the small animal internists have very complicated medical histories. These are the patients with multiple endocrine disorders, especially senior dogs, and some patients come to this service because they need a more intense medical work-up than what their regular veterinarian can provide. Each student is put in charge of one or two patients. We are responsible for examining them, collecting their medical histories, organizing their information into detailed medical notes, and then reporting back to the clinicians in charge. It is also our job to contact pet owners, at least twice a day. Most important of all, we need to come up with a plan for these patients. For example, a 10-year-old pug has a history of coughing. He is up to date on his heartworm prevention, and he has a slight heart murmur on his physical exam. His cough is also a honking type of cough. He is still eating and drinking well, and he isn't having any vomiting or diarrhea. What do you do next?

At this point, students need to come up with a plan for diagnostics. Diagnostics provide more information about our patients because there is only so much useful information you can gather from a medical history and an examination. This is especially true because our patients cannot tell us what the problem is, but oh, how I wished that pug could say, "Well, I cough whenever I do this!" In the case of this pug, x-rays of his chest would be useful to help rule out heart disease, lung disease, and a problem called a collapsing trachea. The trachea, or "windpipe," can become narrow or inflexible overtime, contributing to a honking cough in some patients. Alternatively, blood work is also usually recommended to help rule out an infection or an underlying problem with the internal organs. In order to determine if the heart murmur is a problem, additional diagnostics like an electrocardiogram and an echocardiogram would be useful.

Clinical rotations provide other opportunities to learn. Sometimes, neighboring departments will call each other up to say, "Hey, come check out this cool finding!" There are also case rounds in the morning and in the afternoon. Case rounds are when we sit in a room with a large table and discuss cases with our attending clinicians and professors. They ask us questions about the case and might quiz us on what certain clinical signs or lab values mean. In some cases, we had cage-side rounds so that we could look at the patient while discussing him or her. If you've ever stayed at a human hospital, you might notice that your nurses have bedside rounds so that the incoming nurse can get updates on your progress when they come on shift. Cage-side rounds are almost exactly like this.

Each clinical rotation had its own set of requirements. In internal medicine, we had to provide formal presentations on interesting cases that we'd worked on or started up. It is so nerve-wracking to discuss complicated details in front of professors, clinicians, and your fellow classmen! Part of what was so scary for me was that these doctors would ask you questions about your patient, or they might ask you what certain test values could indicate. Although these are important questions that are pertinent to what we need to know as future doctors, it can be embarrassing and discouraging when you get a question wrong. Just remember that we are all students at some point, and things get better as you become more experienced. There were a lot of times where I would reply, "I'm not sure, but I'll look it up and get back to you with an answer."

Many of UF's patients come from very far away. Not every city has access to a specialty hospital with boarded doctors, advanced imaging, and surgical capabilities. We've even had patients come to us from out of state. So where do their owners stay if the patient needs to remain in the hospital for more than a day or two? If owners live an hour or two from UF, many choose to drive back home while others might check into a local hotel. In either case, it is always important for the owners to be well-informed about their animal's progress, so students are tasked with contacting owners at least twice a day. Not only is this a courtesy for the clients, it is also a way for students to hone their communication skills.

Students are also tasked with taking notes for patient medical records. Depending on which department you're in, there are specific templates for discharge instructions. These pages of instructions summarize the patient's history, details about diagnostics, results, information about certain illnesses, and treatment recommendations. Not only do discharge instructions provide clear information about a specific patient, they also provide details about a case to the referring veterinarian. It seems like not very long ago that my name was printed on the "student" line on the bottom of these instructions. Now it still surprises me when I see my name posted in the referring veterinarian heading!

Every department relies on the pharmacy for patient medications. Whether it's an oral pain medication for a cat, an injectable antibiotic for a horse, or fruit-flavored medications for birds, the pharmacy provides a never-ending list of products for our patients. At UF, it is located in between the small and large animal hospitals. Students would bring their written prescriptions (signed by the clinicians) to the pharmacy and then make sure the medications got picked up later on. If you didn't pick up the prescriptions in time, you would be in lots of trouble!

Clinical rotations usually last for two weeks, but some of the more intensive rotations will last for four weeks. Internal medicine is a four-week rotation, as is surgery. If you are tracking small animal medicine, i.e., you intend to graduate and be a small animal veterinarian, your small animal internal med and surgery rotations will last four weeks each. Large animal internal med and surgery are also requirements, but small animal tracks only require two weeks of each. If you are tracking large animal medicine, it is the inverse of these.

Somehow, I survived my small animal internal medicine rotation, and I moved onto additional clinical rotations like cardiology, neurology, and radiology. My small animal surgery rotation was broken up into two phases: soft tissue surgery for two weeks, followed by two weeks of orthopedic surgery. The surgery rotations were very different from being on the ground level of the hospital and in rounds rooms, because the majority of your time was spent in the vast operating rooms on the second floor.

Most general practicing hospitals have one operating room, aka surgical suite. UF's Small Animal Hospital has more than ten of these rooms! I was definitely out of my element because

I had never seen surgery this close before, and most of the procedures are different from the routine spays and neuters that I had seen as a veterinary technician. Some procedures were exceptionally complicated, and orthopedic surgeries like knee and hip surgery would take hours for the doctors to complete. Students with surgical patients would help prep them for surgery by contacting the anesthesia student and coordinating lab work, intravenous catheter placement, and paperwork. Then the surgical student would follow the patient into the operating room, stay with them in recovery, and follow them down to whichever ward they were scheduled to stay in. Students also called owners the moment surgery started and ended.

Even though this rotation cemented the idea that I am not a fan of surgical procedures, I had a lot of fun, and I felt comfortable with the knowledge I had acquired. I knew that I wanted to focus on general practice work, just like the vets with whom I'd worked. This is probably why Primary Care and Dentistry became my favorite rotation of all!

I remember thinking that this rotation would probably be like all of the others. I knew that I'd be a terrified student, worried about making mistakes or calling out the wrong answers during rounds. If I didn't know the answers, I'd make up for it by rushing to find the answer while also putting in a lot of effort to help other students and provide excellent patient care. I steeled myself for moments of disappointment in myself, but instead, I was pleasantly surprised.

On the first day, one of the doctors was discussing a patient with me. It was a small dog who had come in for his vaccines. The owner was concerned about dirt in the dog's ears, and he had been shaking his head a lot. The lead doctor then asked me, "What would you like to do for this dog's ears?" I remembered that the doctors at my job would collect a sample of the debris from inside of the ears and then roll them out in a thin layer onto a microscope slide. From there, the slide is heat-fixed, stained, and then analyzed under a microscope. This process is called an ear cytology. So when I squeaked out my answer, that I would recommend an ear cytology, my lead doctor replied, "Excellent!"

Suddenly, everything clicked for me. The things that I had learned in the classroom, the things I'd learned in earlier clinical rotations, and the things I'd learned as a vet tech—all of it put me in a position where I felt like I knew what I was doing. I correctly answered a question, and it was one that made complete sense to me! I had already had the idea of working in small animal general practice after graduation, and the confidence and excitement that I felt during the Primary Care and Dentistry rotation really drove the point home for me.

There were lots of fun elements on these rotations, but Integrative Medicine was the most fun because, at times, it didn't feel like work at all. In Integrative Medicine, vets utilize many other elements of medicine to help patients. This includes acupuncture, cold laser therapy, physical therapy, swim therapy, and use of an underwater treadmill. At UF, the hydrotherapy equipment is housed behind large glass windows that look out upon a small courtyard with grass and sunlight. I loved to help the treadmill patients because I often needed to take off my shoes and socks, roll up my pant legs, and walk in the water to help support the dog or cat patient as they exercised. There is something relaxing about the feel of the water and the view from the windows. Every session seemed to go by quickly. I never did get to put on waders and help patients with swim therapy in the great big infinity pool, but maybe I will have a chance someday.

The anesthesia department at UF is located on the second floor, just outside of the operating rooms. This makes it easier to anesthetize patients and then roll the tables and anesthesia carts into these rooms. However, there were times when you would need to anesthetize a patient on the second floor and then hop on the elevator to get to the ground floor. Some of the more advanced imaging like CT scanning took place in a room located in the Large Animal Hospital, so you would have to travel a great distance with your sleeping patient. Despite the worn-out shoes, Anesthesia was a lot of fun because you worked with all the departments, and no two cases were alike. You also learned where all the departments are located because your patient caseload would be greatly varied. Sometimes, Anesthesia students would tag another in on a case so that the first student could get to lunch or go watch an interesting procedure.

Zoo Med was another fun rotation because you never worked with less than three different species a day. We took care of injured wildlife like gopher tortoises and birds of prey. We treated pets owned by clients and animals owned by zoos. The most exciting cases would be the ones where a full-grown alligator or a tiger needed to be anesthetized for special testing. You would get a lot of stares from people in the hospital as you walked down the hall proudly pushing the cart for one of these patients! In the second week of Zoo Med, we went on field trips to visit zoos and wildlife facilities in order to care for some of the animals there.

Food Animal Medicine is one of the rotations that surprised me. As a small animal student, I didn't think I was going to enjoy farm work. We had to get up *extremely* early to get to the farm by 5 AM, meaning that I was up and getting ready around 3 or 4 AM. However, I had a lot of fun hopping into a truck with some of my closest classmates and then driving to a farm in the pitch dark. We arrived at many of these places as the sun was rising, which was always a beautiful sight. There was something peaceful and serene about the mornings. Even the patients who were awaiting their vaccines and exams did not fuss or fight. I was a little sad to wrap up this rotation but walked away with a newfound appreciation for early morning drives and cooperative cows!

Clinical rotations continued over the summer and into the fall semester. By December, the junior year of clinics wrapped up, and we tagged in the next class of seniors so they could start their final round of clinical rotations. We juniors had a short break before heading back into the classroom in the spring semester. I remember that, by this point, much of what I had learned in my first two years had really connected with what I saw on my clinical rotations. This made the end of junior year much easier than the first two years of coursework, and I made it to my final summer vacation as a veterinary student. Students could focus on externships, which are programs that are meant to help further their work experience. I did an externship at the same hospital where I worked as a vet tech, but it was strange being on the other side!

During the summer break of junior year, students also begin prepping for the scariest vet school experience of all: board exams. It isn't enough to just graduate with your four-year veterinary medical degree. Students who attend accredited veterinary schools in the United States must take a grueling exam called the North American Veterinary Licensing Examination, or NAVLE. It is a standardized test that consists of 360 questions broken up into six blocks. The NAVLE can take anywhere from 6.5 to 7.5 hours to complete. This test covers information from all aspects of veterinary medicine, and it is considered the biggest hurdle for all veterinary students. There are other requirements for students of non-accredited and international veterinary schools who wish to practice in the United States. Not only do they need to take the NAVLE, they also need to obtain certification through the PAVE (Program for the Assessment of Veterinary Education Equivalence).

The fall semester of senior year involves being back in the classroom again. The courses, however, are more in tune with your track as a veterinary student. This means that small animal students mostly take small animal courses, and large animal students mostly take large animal courses. There are also more elective courses rather than required ones. In the evenings, professors and doctors would volunteer their time and go over information that they felt would be covered by the NAVLE's questions. These evening sessions were voluntary but very useful, and many students were in attendance.

There are also companies like Zuku and VetPrep who sell software that goes over sample questions from the NAVLE. Some questions are pretty straightforward with only one or two sentences that ask about the definition of something. Other questions are lengthy and provide case information about a patient. The lengthier questions usually ask for answers about recommended diagnostics or what comes next, but the biggest laugh is when a question goes into detail about a patient and ends up asking about something totally different!

I was always a night owl in vet school. I would stay up very late and squeeze as much information into my brain as I could, but with the amount of information you need to know, this is not feasible or sustainable. It's probably why I ran into trouble with the Academic Advancement Committee earlier in my career, so I really don't recommend late-night cram sessions. For the NAVLE, I made a point of going over the important information on various subjects, but I divided up the subjects amongst different days. For example, I focused on cardiology one night and then internal medicine the next. I was very lucky to have the Big Sister that I did because she gave me her giant binder of prep work and questions for when she'd taken the NAVLE the previous year.

The NAVLE is offered at testing centers twice a year, in the fall and in the spring. Most of my classmates decided to sit for the NAVLE around the November/December cycle, including myself. We registered in the summertime and then picked the dates for when we would take it, while a few other classmates opted to take more time to prepare and planned for it in the springtime, just before graduation. My day to take the test was November 20th because I wanted to be finished with it before the Thanksgiving break.

They say that you should avoid studying the night before. This is sound advice because you really should focus on trying to relax that night. But since this is the most difficult test you'll take in your life, how can anyone really relax? I tried to get to bed early that night but ended up tossing and turning for two hours. After a sleep aid and some meditation-type music, I was able to fall asleep.

I'm pretty sure that I looked at a few more NAVLE notes on the morning of test day, just to make sure that I remembered things like mathematical formulas and calculations for medications and fluid rates. I brought some snacks and drinks with me to keep in the locker at the testing center. You are permitted to take a 15-minute break in between each of the six exam blocks, so it was useful to have these items handy. Since most testing centers get a little chilly, they encouraged us to bring a jacket, too. You also needed to have your photo identification handy.

I felt pretty confident as I sat through two straight blocks of questions. I took a 15-minute break and then went back to the next two blocks. I was getting a little less confident and *very* tired as I pushed through them. I made sure to take another 15-minute break because I knew my stamina was draining. The test screen and questions in the final two blocks were a blur because I knew I was hitting my absolute limit. It was a relief when I hit the last question of the sixth block, but I still felt completely exhausted. I managed to finish the NAVLE in about five hours, but I was pretty sure that my soul left my body at some point. To help brighten my spirits, I went out to eat with some of my classmates who sat for the test during the same session as me. We each felt a bit nervous about not knowing if we had passed or failed, but we celebrated nonetheless!

There are a few students who fail the NAVLE when they take it for the first time. It is possible to retake the exam, but there are limits to how many times you can take it. Each of us worried about possibly failing the NAVLE and dreaded the possibility of having to retake it. We would not find out our pass/fail status until February which was still three months away. By January, we seniors were back on the clinic floor and starting our final rotations.

I was in the middle of my Emergency and Critical Care rotation when word got out one February morning that the NAVLE scores were posted to the website portal. I can't tell you how many times I'd logged in each day prior to that to see if scores had been posted, but rumors indicated that it would be sometime in the beginning or middle of February. I fumbled with my fingers as I tried to type the website name into the internet browser, and then I logged in. My first impression was that I had failed because there was a rectangle in the middle of the screen that was a brick-red color, but I then noticed that it said "PASS" in white lettering. Words cannot express the immense relief I felt as the months of worry and self-doubt dissolved away.

Many of our classmates and rotation-mates were excitedly calling and texting one another, and it was great hearing about each classmate who passed the NAVLE. However, I started to worry about the students I hadn't heard from yet. Had they failed? It turns out that a couple of them did, and I felt so bad for them because I know that they put a lot of effort into studying and preparing, probably even more than I had! These students were completely dejected, but I'm happy to report that they all went on to pass the NAVLE the second time that they took it in the springtime. If you find yourself in their situation, give yourself a good seven days to forgive yourself, bolster your confidence, and move on.

I was a different student in my senior year of clinics compared to my sophomore/junior year transition. So much of what I had learned was now memorable and easy to apply to my cases. The questions that were asked in case rounds were no longer scary or difficult, and I didn't have that deer-in-the-headlights look when professors would grill me on certain topics. I was on track to graduate and was getting increasingly excited as the days went by.

Before graduating, students need to know their plans for when they've finished school. Most students intend to start practicing right away, while some consider internships. Internships can offer more real-world experience under the supervision of other veterinarians, and they are optional for students considering general practice. If you are considering specializing in a certain area, and you plan on applying for a residency program, most schools require an internship before you can apply for a residency. Since I had no plans for specialized medicine, I chose to go straight into practice after graduation.

Some schools will help you work on your résumé so that you can apply for jobs while you are still a student. I planned on applying to the same corporate small animal hospital that I had worked for as a veterinary technician, but my current hospital wasn't hiring any doctors at the time. I talked with the medical director for the neighboring market and had a job interview at one of the locations in Central Florida. She offered me a job, and I was able to shadow some of the staff at different locations that were hiring. After I went back home and discussed the job offer with my husband, we decided that we would move to Orlando after graduation so that I could start work in Central Florida right away.

During some of my free time in the final semester, we made trips to Orlando to secure housing that would be close to my new hospital. We found an older home to rent, one where the landlord said that it was okay to bring our many dogs and cats to live with us. This eased our minds, considering most rentals only permit one or two pets. I was set to start my new job in June, which was only a couple of months away.

The final week of your clinical year as a senior is such an exciting time. Graduation is just around the corner, and you're almost an official doctor! But one of the other things I really enjoyed was when the newly coated sophomore class came onto the clinic floor. I can remember being as scared as they were, but I must have been a comfort to some of them because when it came time to figure out which student would be assigned to shadow which senior, I had three descend upon me all at once! I had three students shadowing me that week, and they all did a great job learning the tasks for the rotation.

I don't think any of us were able to focus on that final Friday. The seniors are officially dismissed by noon, and there is a big send-off from the professors and hospital staff. Most of us got together for a pool party afterward (this is Florida, after all), and some of us said our final goodbyes leading up to graduation.

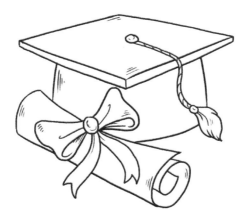

Hearing "doctor" in front of your name for the first time is one of the strangest sensations. I have vivid memories of that moment when my name was called, when I walked across the stage at graduation and received my diploma. My whole family was there for me, even relatives from up north. I felt so supported and loved because this large, loud group of my favorite people came out to see me graduate. It was one of the best days of my life, and I still carry everyone's love and support with me every day. I consider myself quite lucky, and I never thought that my heart would feel so full once I entered this profession.

CHAPTER 10

THE DIFFICULTIES OF PRACTICING VETERINARY MEDICINE

I was fortunate to attend veterinary school with some of the best doctors that I know. Each of us has different opinions regarding the career path we've chosen. For me, I loved my time as a student, and I enjoy my job as a small animal veterinarian. It may be disheartening to learn that there are lots of veterinarians who do not feel the same way. When asked if they would be okay with attending vet school all over again, some say that they would choose a totally different career path if given the choice.

The life of a veterinarian isn't always easy. You've probably heard us say that it's not just about snuggling puppies and kittens each day. We choose this career because we love animals. We want to help those who are helpless, and we want to help the people who care for them. However, there are many hardships that veterinarians face every day, and for some, they can seem insurmountable.

Being a new graduate is difficult. Even though you have this terrific amount of knowledge in your head, there are moments where it is hard to apply what you've learned to a real-life situation. When you don't know the answer to a question, a student can look up the answer or check their notes. But when you don't know how to help your patient, you feel enormously guilty because this pet's life is in your hands. You start to fill up with self-doubt and wonder if the patient would be better off seeing a more experienced veterinarian. You start to think that you're not cut out for this field and that you are incompetent. And even when you're doing a great job, you don't see yourself in that light. This is known as imposter syndrome, and it affects many new graduates in medical professions.

When humans are sick and need to go to an emergency room or call poison control, there is government funding in place to cover the bill up front so that an empty wallet doesn't mean the difference between life or death for people. This is not the case for veterinary medicine. Small animal hospitals and emergency rooms are businesses that do not receive government funding, which means that most pet owners are expected to pay for tests and services before they are rendered. If these businesses do not earn enough money to pay for electricity, rent, products, and staff, then these businesses shut down. But this also puts veterinarians in a hard spot because there are so many animals who need our help, and there are owners who simply cannot afford tests or treatments.

There will be times where you have a patient that has a serious illness, one that might be treatable with several days of hospital care, antibiotics, intravenous fluids, and other treatments. For example, you may have a very young but lethargic puppy present to you with dehydration and black, tarry stool. If he hasn't had vaccines yet, you might wonder if he has parvovirus, which is a nasty intestinal virus that can cause death without aggressive supportive care. The kind of care that this puppy needs will be very expensive, maybe close to $1,000 or more! Pets with insurance from independent companies might be covered for these events, but very few pets have pet insurance, including this puppy. This owner has just lost their job and has been declined for special health care credit through a third-party company. What do you do when the owner of this puppy says that they cannot afford treatment?

In situations where animals are very sick or suffering, humane euthanasia is recommended because it is our job as veterinarians to ease suffering for animals. Euthanasia is when a veterinarian administers high doses of an anesthetic drug so that the animal passes away. It causes the heart to stop, and breathing ceases, but it is like falling asleep and is not painful or stressful. In the case of this puppy who is in pain and very lethargic, it is likely that he will pass away without treatment. This is cruel to the puppy and to the owner who will have to watch him waste away. Even though this puppy could improve with treatment, euthanasia is a fair decision.

There may be many more situations where you have a patient with something manageable or treatable, but then the owner may have financial hardship, or the pet's quality of life is too poor to continue. Veterinarians have to make decisions like this every day. What is even worse is that sometimes these sad situations are squeezed in between normal appointments. So you might have to say goodbye to a wonderful old patient one moment and then go meet a new puppy patient a few minutes later. Having to move from a sad situation to a happy one in such a short period of time causes outrageous emotional whiplash. Even if a veterinarian looks well put together in one moment, they could be dealing with a mixed bag of emotions beneath the surface.

Veterinary medicine can be a thankless job, and we are always grateful for the people who take the time to say that we make a difference. But not everyone looks upon veterinarians favorably. In the moments where we cannot help a patient without funds, some pet owners think of us as being cruel or heartless. If we're in a rush on a busy day, we are perceived as being emotionless or not caring enough about a patient. It only takes a few minutes to make an impression on someone, and if we're not extremely careful, we might end up with complaints or bad reviews posted online.

"If you really loved animals, you would help me."

"If you cared, you wouldn't suggest euthanasia for my pet."

It is important to recognize that when people say things like this, you are being subjected to abuse. Instead of taking responsibility for their pet's health, they are fixing the blame on you because you aren't able to assume financial responsibility for their pet's illness. But what can you say to someone in this situation that will make everyone feel better? Sometimes there just isn't an answer, and you cannot fix everything. Emotional abuse and helplessness are a part of what contributes to mental health issues such as burnout and compassion fatigue.

Burnout is the term for the mental and physical exhaustion that results from chronic stress in the workplace. Burnout is very common in veterinary medicine, particularly among small animal vets, because there is immense pressure to see many patients each day. Not only does the pressure apply to helping patients and clients, it also applies to the financial side of keeping your business afloat. Eventually, burnout can contribute to compassion fatigue, which is when a veterinarian starts to feel less empathy and compassion toward people and patients. This stems from continued stress and mental exhaustion from the demands of veterinary medicine. Compassion fatigue is also part of why the suicide rate for veterinarians in the United States is higher than in any other profession.

Veterinarians are great at taking care of their animal patients, but they are probably the worst at taking care of themselves, including me! It is important for veterinarians to recognize signs of burnout and compassion fatigue in their colleagues and in themselves so that the appropriate action can be taken. Focusing on mindfulness and meditation can help strengthen your frame of mind, and activities outside of veterinary medicine can help you to relax or unwind. Therapy can help veterinarians who deal with severe anxiety, depression, or even thoughts of suicide. Regular exercise, healthy eating habits, and at least seven or eight hours of sleep can keep you physically healthy.

Over time, it becomes easier to leave work at work and focus on being not-a-doctor at home. There are times on busy days where I almost get sick of hearing the sound of my name being repeated. "Dr. Irish, we need you in the treatment area!" Just hearing my first name being spoken at home makes me feel human again. Part of self-preservation in this field is being able to leave the doctor version of yourself back at work. Sure, there may be situations where an animal needs help on the side of the road, or a random high school classmate messages you at 2 AM because their pet is sick. In time, it becomes easier to act when and if you are able. If you need to heal, you learn to set firm boundaries. This is one of the most important aspects of self-care.

Human doctors go through the same rigorous schooling as veterinarians, but human doctors tend to earn more than double what a veterinarian earns. This can make it very difficult to pay off student loans that were necessary to pay for vet school tuition. In cases like mine, additional loans were necessary to cover the cost of living in a college town because I was not able to keep regular work hours while in school, and my husband could only earn so much to support us. For students that attend vet school out of state or internationally, their tuition and cost of living will be even higher. Once you've graduated from vet school, the interest starts to accrue on these student loans, and the monthly payments can be double what it costs for a mortgage on a home!

The most obvious difficulty in practicing veterinary medicine is that our patients cannot talk to us. If they could tell us what hurts and where, our lives would be so much easier! Veterinarians must rely on a pet owner's descriptions and medical history for their pet. Physical examinations and diagnostics are just pieces of a very large puzzle, and sometimes it takes a lot of pieces before you can get a clear picture.

Some test results can appear normal even in the face of something bad lurking beneath the surface. A good example is when a dog's bloodwork looks normal, but there is a cancerous tumor growing on his liver. Sometimes we might exhaust all of our test options and find nothing. In instances where owners cannot afford testing, veterinarians must make an educated guess about what could be happening. We rely on the mantra that "common things happen commonly" and start from there. If a patient doesn't respond to initial therapy, we have them follow up for another exam and then try something else. This will work some of the time, but it can be frustrating when it doesn't.

If you ever find yourself in a situation where you are doubting your abilities, take a moment to reflect on how far you've come. All of your schooling and prior experiences have brought you to this point. You may not be able to fix everything or make everyone happy, but there are a lot of people (and patients!) who think that you're the best doctor around. Remember the ones who make *you* happy and always keep in mind that you make a world of difference. In moments of doubt and worry, take a deep breath and keep moving forward.

CHAPTER 11:

THE PROS OF PRACTICING VETERINARY MEDICINE

It seems easier to remember the moments that cause us worry, stress, or anxiety. Most of us recall our first customer complaints or bad reviews online, and none of us forget the angry clients that yell at us or chew us out over the phone. These are problems that most people face at work, but they are rare occurrences. There are many more positive aspects to the work that people do each day, and veterinary medicine is loaded with them.

The majority of veterinarians choose this field because they want to help animals, especially those of us who had pets growing up. I had so many different animals as a child, and I grew up with a very loving Beagle named Zoe. I wanted to be able to help all of my pets, which is probably what propelled me toward a career in veterinary medicine, and my Zoe's heart disease in her senior years stimulated my curiosity for all things cardiology. Once I became a veterinary technician and then a veterinarian, I was able to take my own pet ownership experiences and apply them to situations where other owners would find themselves. These shared experiences help me to connect with pet owners, and in a way, they help me to practice better medicine. I've also made a lot of close friends in this field, from clients to coworkers.

I'm a very extroverted person, which means that I'm outgoing and love socialization. Extroverts also tend to draw energy from the people around them, so I really enjoy my interactions with coworkers and clients every day. Talking comes very naturally to me, and over time, I've become very skilled at communicating with owners. I like being able to take complicated medical information and "translate" it for them, and I really love talking to owners about how great their pets are. Sometimes, we'll even swap stories about our own pets, which makes for very fun (and funny!) conversations.

The biggest pro to working in this field is that I do get to snuggle puppies and kittens from time to time. It's so fun to start out with a very young animal and then watch them grow with each appointment. Sometimes, I will look at the appointment schedule on our work computers, see a patient name, and remember what they looked like when they were younger. Inevitably, I end up surprised at check-in to see how big they've gotten!

My favorite appointments are the dogs and cats that come in wearing articles of clothing. Some come in wearing shirts with bright colors or funny sayings. The pets with neck ties and bowties on their collars always look so professional and dapper. A favorite patient of mine would come in with a bright yellow raincoat during the wettest days. Another favorite patient always has different colored tutus stitched onto her harness.

I have a pretty sharp memory, so I can easily recall the different quirks and mannerisms for most of my patients. A fear-aggressive German Shepherd patient of mine will only let us give him his vaccinations if he can sit on the soft chairs in a specific exam room. One cat patient who I see for frequent blood checks needs to have his stuffed toy with him at all times. A very timid but sweet Golden Retriever insists on shaking my hand or "giving paw" whenever I examine him. A favorite Labrador mix patient would sniff her owner's hair every time she came home from her bakery job, so every time I examined this dog, I would have to get down on the floor and let her sniff my hair as a greeting!

For most veterinarians, coworkers become your work-family. I work with other doctors, veterinary technicians, receptionists, and support staff. Even the busiest days can be fun and rewarding when you are part of a great team! I've made lots of close friendships along the way, and you never know who you'll run into again because the veterinary community is quite small, meaning that everyone seems to know everyone. With the right kinds of relationships in your community, you may be able to call in favors or borrow something from a neighboring hospital if you've run out. I love knowing that there is this wide support system out there for me as a veterinarian and as a member of the community. I've made lots of friends in other medical professions, and we will often ask each other medical questions based on our respective fields of expertise. It's been nice to randomly text my pediatrician or my dentist, and I don't mind answering any questions they have about their own pets!

Education is a big part of veterinary medicine, and I don't just mean the schooling that got you to this point. My job is to educate clients each day regarding routine care, use of medications, certain diseases, and various dangers or risks for their pets regarding exposure to things like human medications and poisonous plants. I also love teaching new information or concepts to the staff, and even though I'm not crazy about math, I like being able to teach technicians different ways of calculating medication dosages and fluid rates. Sharing new ways of doing things or the latest data from published studies helps to keep me up to date on things as well. I especially love training veterinary students and externs because I remember having fun during my time in vet school, and I want these vets in training to do well and enjoy their time, too.

Like all medical fields, veterinary medicine is constantly changing. There are always new techniques, tests, medications, and treatment methods. Scientific studies are published multiple times a month, and there always seems to be the "latest and greatest" in terms of equipment and products for us to use. To ensure that doctors are being kept up to date on advances in medicine, it is a legal requirement to have a certain number of hours of continuing education every two years. This could mean watching a lecture live online or going to a conference in person and listening to a speaker. For me, I can enjoy these lectures a little more than in vet school because I know that I'm not going to be graded on it afterward. Conferences are also another time to socialize with other vets, support staff, and different product manufacturers and pharmaceutical representatives. It's always exciting to see the newest gadgets and products.

One of the unexpected pros for me was discovering that I could use my medical knowledge for other things besides clinical practice. I've always been pretty strong in verbal and written communication, so when I discovered that various pet-based websites needed veterinarians for medical articles and fact-checking, I was pleasantly surprised. Doing this kind of writing in my spare time has not only allowed me to educate a broader audience, it has also helped to keep my current medical knowledge up to date. When I write research articles on certain topics, I usually find new ways to describe things or new information. Writing even helps me to understand how things work, whereas my prior knowledge of such things was minimal at best. Besides writing, veterinarians can also seek employment in a teaching capacity with vet tech schools and veterinary schools.

Even though veterinarians have a different medical school experience than human doctors, the foundations of our medical knowledge and expertise are identical. This comes in handy in many situations and not just for running all of the medical categories on Jeopardy! Having medical knowledge is useful for understanding how diseases affect humans, how medications work and interact, and knowing the names of various tests and why they are recommended. It also gives me insight into how doctors think and why they might prescribe one test or treatment versus another. In situations where family members have had various medical recommendations, I've been able to decipher medical jargon and explain things in simpler terms for them. When my family members have appointments with their doctors, I am sometimes asked to come with them so that I can explain what is happening and think up some follow-up questions that they might not otherwise think of for clarification.

For me, the positives of veterinary medicine outweigh many of the negatives. Perhaps I'm lucky in that I can take mental breaks from the stressful parts of practicing medicine. Or it might have something to do with my support system. My family and friends are so loving and supportive of me. My mother is so proud of the fact that I'm a doctor, and she talks to her friends about me all the time. My father, who works at an international airport, will strike up conversations with travelers that end in boasting sessions regarding his smart daughter in Central Florida. My husband worked hard to support us while I was in vet school, and he's been my biggest fan for almost two decades. My coworkers know when I'm having a stressful workday and will quickly cheer me up with coffee, snacks, and my favorite music. I have so many lovely clients and patients that I end up seeing at least one of my favorites every single day. On various occasions, people have told me that I saved their best friends, that I made such a difference in their lives, that I gave their pet more time on earth, and that I am a great doctor. I can't think of any other job on this planet that could make my heart feel as full as it does to this day!

CHAPTER 12:

WAYS TO PREPARE FOR A CAREER IN VETERINARY MEDICINE

There are other ways to prepare yourself for a career in veterinary medicine besides focusing on your test scores and work experience. Much of it has to do with your financial preparedness, your mental preparedness, and how you stand out from a crowd of other vet school applicants.

It may sound strange, but the interviewers for vet school want to hear more about what makes you different from everyone else. It's so easy to say that you are passionate about caring for animals because that's how we all feel, and it's probably what drove more than half of us to become veterinarians. But how do you manage your work-life balance? What are other things you enjoy, and how do you recharge your batteries at the end of the day? Do you enjoy swimming or running? Do you have some kind of athletic background or play sports? Or do you simply meditate and attend yoga classes? For me, I picked up ballet shoes at age 20 just because I'd always wanted to dance. I took classes for a few years, even during vet school, but I stopped attending when it was time to focus on studying for the NAVLE. I'll never forget the dance recital that happened after a full night of emergencies during my first clinical rotations. I didn't get any sleep the night before! I went straight to the stage when I was released, and I honestly don't remember most of it. However, my friends who attended assured me that I did well.

Volunteer service is a great way to spend your free time. If you volunteer at an animal hospital or shelter, you will get real experience that can help you for years to come. You can start small with things like cleaning and disinfecting kennels, and you can gradually work up to restraining patients in order to assist vets and vet techs. Volunteering around the community, like in homeless shelters or low-cost care clinics, is very rewarding because you are making a difference for all those around you. During my shelter medicine rotation, we helped at a low-cost animal care clinic called St. Francis House. Owners with strict financial limitations would bring their pets to see us for vaccines and basic care for minor issues like ear and skin infections. It was so heartwarming to help these happy patients, and the gratitude that their owners expressed almost brought tears to my eyes.

Keep in mind that vet school is expensive, as is the cost of living while you're in school. This is especially true if you have to move out of state or outside of the country to attend vet school. Even though my family lived in southwest Florida, I still had to move four hours away to attend the University of Florida. My husband and I found a tiny studio apartment and went with the bare minimum for amenities. We had to secure jobs right away because we had zero money in savings, and neither of our families had the money to send us to college. He and I were the typical college kids in a college town, subsisting on ramen noodles and Hamburger Helper when we could afford it.

I was fortunate to obtain a Bright Futures Scholarship which paid for 75 percent of my state college tuition, which was a huge relief for my mom! I applied for it while I was in high school, and I had the good grades to receive it. Once I used up all of my Bright Futures Scholarship, I was able to apply for the Pell grant, which is a government program that pays for college for students from low-income households. Once I made it up to UF for the rest of my undergraduate career, I had to apply for student loans. Scholarships and grants are yours to keep, and you don't have to pay them back. Loans will gather interest over time, so you end up having to pay back more than you borrowed. If you borrowed a lot, as I needed to do to attend vet school and live in Gainesville, you will end up with a huge sum of money to pay back.

Student loans are still a large problem for many students, not just those of us in veterinary medicine. Repayment programs are helpful for people like me who have a high debt-to-income ratio. This means that my student loan debt is much larger than what I could afford to pay back based on my earnings. Repayment programs make the monthly payments more affordable for people in my situation, and some of this debt gets forgiven at the end of a certain time period. However, if I don't work for the government or work in underprivileged areas, I will owe taxes on the amount of money that is forgiven. This can be a huge sum of money, anywhere from $50,000 and up.

If at all possible, take as little loan money as you can. If you are able to get a job now, save that money for your college education. You can add it to what your parents have saved for you, if anything. Apply for as many scholarships and grants as you can. If you're able to stay at home for college, you will save a lot on living expenses, but if this is not possible, consider living with a roommate who can split the cost of an apartment and the amenities with you. State college tuition is much less expensive than university tuition, but check with your vet school to see which course credits they will accept from a state college level.

Make sure that you read up on all the fine print when it comes to college, so that you won't lose any credits if you have to transfer from a state college to a university. Check to see what requirements are necessary so that you aren't missing any items by the time you have to apply. Try to get all of your applications and letters of recommendation in as early as you can so that you won't miss any deadlines. If you could use some help boosting your grades, try studying with some friends or working with a tutor.

CHAPTER 13:

LOOKING BACK ON THE YEARS

I've been a part of the veterinary field for the past 16 years, and I've been a veterinarian for seven of them. If you could go back in time and tell me that I would be a doctor today, I probably wouldn't believe you! It seemed like a simple enough idea when I was discussing my future career with that high school counselor. But when the factors started to pile up—the distance to the school from my home, the amount of extra schooling, the cost, the rates of acceptance of applicants—I really started to doubt myself. I'd always been a pretty smart student, one that would sit down and get all my homework done the moment that I got home, one that didn't need to study too much before an exam, and yet the things that made me remarkable suddenly seemed unremarkable when compared to the outstanding backgrounds of other vet school hopefuls.

On that first day of UF undergrad in 2006, I had been so excited and optimistic knowing that my first class, Animal Sciences, was my intro to the vet school track because it was one of the requirements for UF's vet school. Also, I had yet to take any courses that exclusively focused on animals, and so I was eager to learn everything the lecturers had to offer. However, as the professors introduced themselves to the class of 200 or so students, they made a point of having us look around the room.

"Look at all of the people around you," one of the professors said. "The majority of you have an interest in becoming a veterinarian, and most of you won't make it into the program."

As if that wasn't enough to deflate my lofty ambitions, the entire course focused on farm animals and things like milk yield from cows and beef production. These were things I had zero interest in, and perhaps I was a little naïve in thinking that the course would be about dogs and cats. But I did learn a lot, and I made some great friends in that first class.

Much of the rest of my college experience was like my first introduction to animal sciences. Whenever I had an idea about something going one way, it went in a completely different direction. When I thought I could wrap up my bachelor's degree in one year, I needed to take a second year due to the drop in transferred credits from state college. When I didn't get into vet school on my first try, I ended up doing a year in the public health college at UF for graduate-level courses. I didn't get into vet school after my second try, but then that fateful phone call from the associate dean changed everything. I had a setback when I had to go before the Academic Advancement Committee, but I ended up being able to dig my heels in and work harder for the following semester. When I thought I was floundering in my clinical rotations, I was able to make up for my nervousness with perseverance, patient care, and good teamwork.

All of my experiences, the good and the bad, got me to where I am today. I am a doctor of veterinary medicine. I am still that nervous yet excitable student who works hard to learn as much as I can about my patients. With time, patience, effort, and support, I've become comfortable in my medical knowledge and have the skills to do well no matter where I practice. I've even been able to branch out and focus on a writing career on the side.

The bottom line is that there are going to be setbacks on your journey, and you probably won't follow the exact track that you have planned in your mind. Everyone's path to veterinary medicine is so different, and when you ask them, it usually isn't how they expected it would be. There are plenty of vets who hit the pause button on schooling and focused on other careers first. Some vets ended up going to vet schools that weren't their first, second, or even third choice. These schools were out of state or even located in other countries. Some vets will start out tracking one area of medicine but then completely change course at the end. This happens with a lot of zoo medicine vets because the field is very small and competitive. It also happens with large animal vets because of the demands of mobile practice, and many choose to switch to small animal medicine later on.

Keep in mind that you won't foresee every setback, but you can do your best and plan for some of them. Always try to focus on the good things around you, and remember how far you've come in this process. It's very rare for people to tell you that you're doing a great job. During my journey to vet school, no one ever really came out and stated that I was competitive enough to be applying, that I had what it takes to be a veterinarian. But I did have support from friends and family, and when I actively sought feedback from people like the associate dean of the vet school, I was told that I *am* good enough. Receiving this kind of feedback will give you the drive to keep going, even in those moments when it doesn't seem like you'll get to be what you want to be.

If you're interested in becoming a veterinarian, you are already a caring and compassionate person, and you're probably super smart! The world needs more people like that, and veterinary medicine definitely needs more doctors with these character traits. There are so many animals out there that need your help, and you can make a world of difference for more than just your patients.

I hope that you've enjoyed reading this book. Good luck to you in your future endeavors, and I can't wait to work with you in the field someday!

Made in the USA
Middletown, DE
04 December 2022

17058101R00070